Psychiatry
at a Glance

D1354846

This title is also available as an e-book.
For more details, please see
www.wiley.com/buy/9781119129677
or scan this QR code:

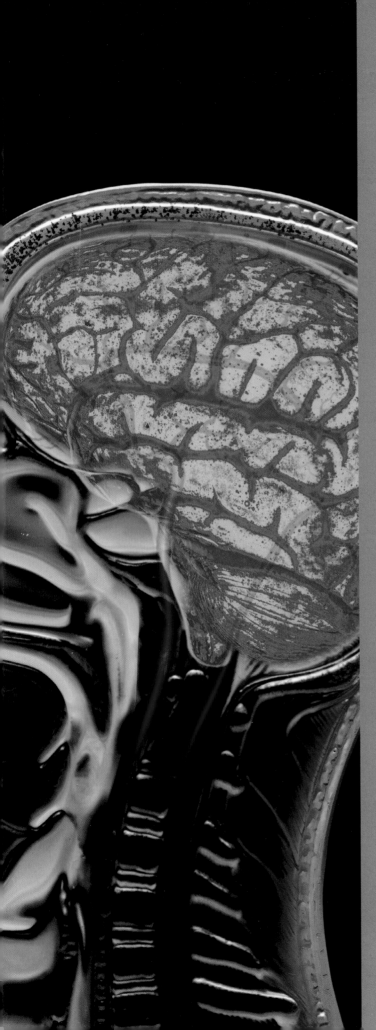

Psychiatry
at a Glance

Sixth Edition

Cornelius Katona

Medical Director
Helen Bamber Foundation;
Honorary Professor
Division of Psychiatry
University College London

Claudia Cooper

Clinical Reader in Old Age Psychiatry
University College London;
Honorary Consultant Psychiatrist
Camden and Islington NHS Foundation Trust

Mary Robertson

Emeritus Professor in Neuropsychiatry
University College London;
Visiting Professor and Honorary Consultant
St George's Hospital and Medical School,
London;
Honorary Professor
Department of Psychiatry
University of Cape Town, South Africa

WILEY Blackwell

Registered office: John Wiley & Sons, Ltd, The Atrium, Southern Gate, Chichester, West Sussex, PO19 8SQ, UK

Editorial offices: 9600 Garsington Road, Oxford, OX4 2DQ, UK
The Atrium, Southern Gate, Chichester, West Sussex, PO19 8SQ, UK
350 Main Street, Malden, MA 02148-5020, USA

For details of our global editorial offices, for customer services and for information about how to apply for permission to reuse the copyright material in this book please see our website at www.wiley.com/wiley-blackwell

Library of Congress Cataloging-in-Publication Data
Katona, C. L. E. (Cornelius L. E.), 1954- , author.
  Psychiatry at a glance / Cornelius Katona, Claudia Cooper, Mary Robertson. – Sixth edition.
    p. ; cm. – (At a glance)
  Includes bibliographical references and index.
  ISBN 978-1-119-12967-7 (pbk.)
  I. Cooper, Claudia, author.   II. Robertson, Mary M., author.   III. Title.   IV. Series: At a glance series (Oxford, England)
  [DNLM: 1. Mental Disorders.   2. Psychiatry. WM 140]
  RC454
  616.89–dc23
                                                                                    2015024744
A catalogue record for this book is available from the British Library.

Wiley also publishes its books in a variety of electronic formats. Some content that appears in print may not be available in electronic books.

Cover image: © Don Farrall/Getty Images

Set in 9.5/11.5pt Minion Pro by Aptara Inc., New Delhi, India
Printed and bound in Singapore by Markono Print Media Pte Ltd

1   2016

Contents

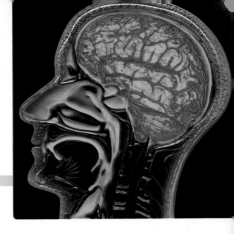

Preface

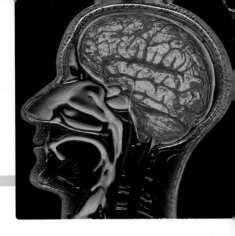

We are delighted that medical students, psychiatrists and GPs in training and other mental health professionals (as well as their trainers) continue to benefit from the concise summary of key practical information about the practice of psychiatry which *Psychiatry at a Glance* provides. We have updated the sixth edition to ensure that it is up to date with regard to the fifth edition of the *Diagnostic and Statistical Manual of Mental Disorders* and with current National Institute of Health and Care Excellence (NICE) guidelines.

We would like to thank Philippa Katona and Mike Carless for their continuing patience and support.

Cornelius Katona
Claudia Cooper
Mary Robertson

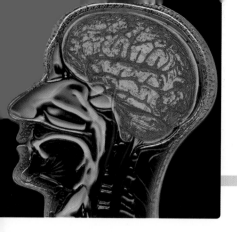

Contributors to Chapter 44

Peter Bazzana
RPN, BHSc (Nursing), M. Suicidology, Member MHRT
Lecturer, New South Wales Institute of Psychiatry,
Sydney, Australia

Valsamma Eapen
MBBS, DPM, PhD, FRCPsych, FRANZCP
Chair of Infant Child and Adolescent Psychiatry,
University of New South Wales
Head, Academic Unit of Child Psychiatry, South Western
Sydney LHD, Sydney, Australia

Ian Ellis-Jones
BA, LLB, LLM, PhD, Dip Relig Stud
Solicitor of the Supreme Court of New South Wales
and the High Court of Australia
Lecturer, New South Wales Institute of Psychiatry,
Sydney, Australia

About the Companion Website

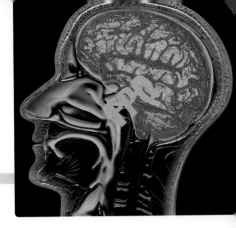

Don't forget to visit the companion website for this book:

www.ataglanceseries.com/psychiatry

There you will find valuable material designed to enhance your learning, including:

- Interactive case studies
- Downloadable illustrations

Scan this QR code to visit the companion website:

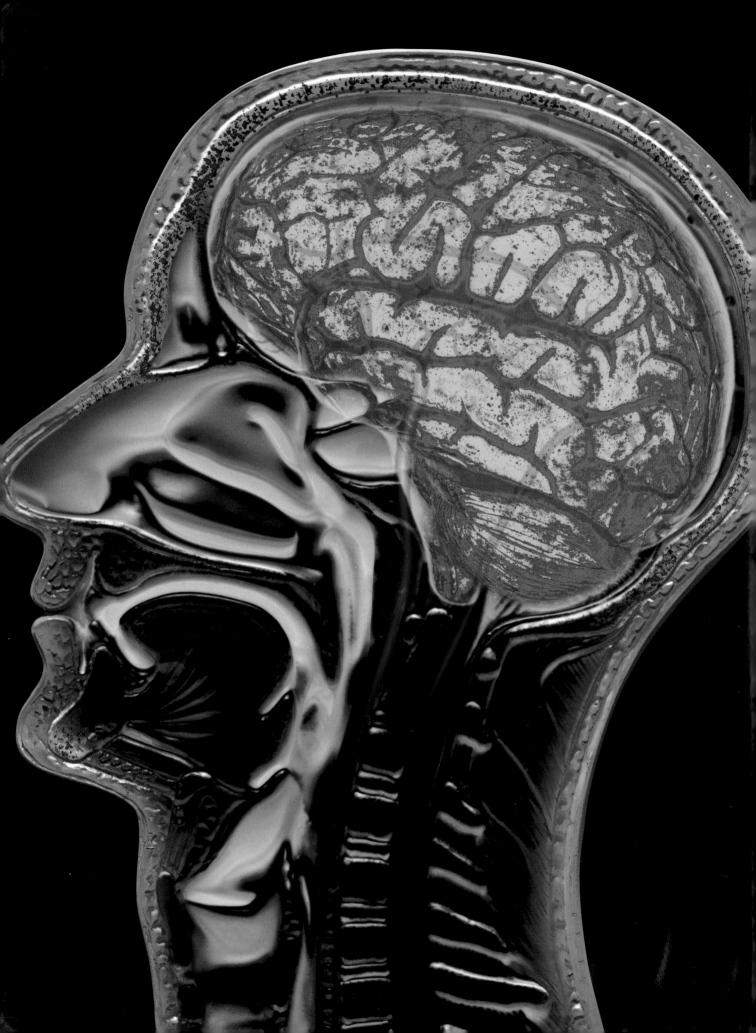

Assessment and Management

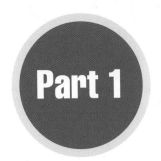

Part 1

Chapters

1 Psychiatric History

An example psychiatric history

Introduction and presenting complaint: Mr John Smith is a 36-year-old Caucasian man, a mechanic, admitted to Florence Ward three days ago after police detained him on Section 136 for acting bizarrely in the street. He is now on Section 2. He thinks his neighbours are plotting to kill him.

History of presenting complaint: Mr Smith last felt free from worry four months ago. Since witnessing his neighbour staring at him, he has believed this neighbour and his wife are intercepting his mail, using a machine so no one can tell that the letters have been opened. He sees red cars outside, which he thinks the neighbours use to monitor his movements. After an altercation on the street three days ago in which he accused these neighbours of pumping gas into his flat, he has believed that they want to kill him or force him to move out so that they can purchase the property. He denies low mood. He cannot rule out the possibility he might defend himself against the neighbours but denies specific plans to retaliate. He denies hearing the neighbours or others talking about him or feeling that they can control him or his thoughts. He has been sleeping poorly. His appetite is reasonable.

Collateral history: Mrs Smith confirmed that her husband had been very preoccupied for the past month with worries about the neighbours intercepting mail and pumping gas into the flat. She witnessed the recent altercation in which her husband was verbally but not physically aggressive to the neighbours. The neighbours are a retired couple who are polite and considerate. Mr Smith has become withdrawn, staying mostly in the kitchen, the only room he believes is 'safe'. He has been hostile to his wife at times this week, which is unusual. This occurred when she questioned his beliefs. He has never threatened her or their daughter.

Past psychiatric history: Mr Smith has seen a psychiatrist once before, aged 8, when he was diagnosed with 'emotional problems'. His GP diagnosed depression when he was 24 and prescribed fluoxetine, which he never took. He believes he was depressed for a couple of years in his mid-20s but denies mental health problems since then. No previous psychiatric admissions. He has never taken medication for mental illness.

Past medical/surgical history: Mild asthma. Nil else of note.

Drug history and allergies: No current medication. No known allergies.

Family history: When Mr Smith was 28, his father died from lung cancer aged 60. His mother and brother, who is eight years younger, live nearby. Both are well, in regular contact and supportive. No known family psychiatric history.

Personal history – early life and development: Normal vaginal delivery, no known complications, no developmental delay. Mr Smith lived in the same house in Doncaster throughout his childhood. His father was a shopkeeper, and his mother a housewife. His parents were happily married, and there were no financial problems at home. No childhood abuse.

Educational history: Mr Smith left school at 16 with five GCEs. He had good friends from school. He was often in trouble with his teachers; he was suspended once for cheating in an exam but was never expelled.

Occupational history: On leaving school Mr Smith worked in the family plumbing business for a few years, then trained and worked as a mechanic. He has never been sacked and has been in his current job for three years. He has been on sick leave for the last two weeks because of 'stress'.

Relationship history: Happily married for 10 years. He has one daughter, aged 5, who is well.

Substance use: Mr Smith drinks 30 units of alcohol a week, mainly wine in the evenings. There is no history of alcohol dependence. He has used cannabis regularly in the past (aged 16–28) but no illicit drug use since this time.

Forensic history: Conviction and fine for driving without due care aged 21. No other arrests or convictions.

Social history: Mr Smith owns his three-bedroom detached house. He usually sees his mother, brother and work friends regularly, but not in the past month. No current financial difficulties.

Premorbid personality: Mr Smith described himself as a sociable, calm person who thought the best of people and didn't tend to get into disputes with others until his current difficulties. He is a keen cyclist and member of a local cycling club.

The psychiatric history and mental state assessment (discussed in Chapter 2) are undertaken together in the *psychiatric interview*. This is a critical time for establishing rapport as well as systematically obtaining this information. In this chapter and the next, we present a format for written documentation; greater flexibility is clearly required during the actual interview. You should always do a physical examination too.

Introduction and presenting complaint

• Patient's name, age, occupation, ethnic origin, circumstances of referral (and, in the case of inpatients, whether voluntary or compulsory) and presenting complaint (in the patient's own words).

History of the present illness

• Start with open questions, e.g. 'Can you tell me what has been happening?'
• Establish when the illness first began (and, if a relapsing/remitting illness, when this illness episode began), e.g. 'When did you last feel well?'
• What does the patient think might have caused the illness as a whole or this relapse/recurrence, and what makes it better or worse?
• What has been the effect on daily life/relationships/work?
• Depending on the presenting complaint, you will need to ask follow-up questions about other symptoms to help you make a diagnosis. Your questions should be guided by the diagnostic criteria for

Psychiatry at a Glance, Sixth Edition. Cornelius Katona, Claudia Cooper, Mary Robertson. © 2016 John Wiley & Sons, Ltd. Published 2016 by John Wiley & Sons, Ltd.
Companion website: www.ataglanceseries.com/psychiatry

the individual disorders (discussed in later chapters). For example, if the patient describes feeling anxious, you would ask questions to establish if the anxiety is situational and if panic attacks occur.

• Enquire about mood, sleep and appetite, even if they appear normal, and whether there are risks of harm to self or others (see Chapters 4 and 5).

Especially in psychosis or dementia, the patients' views of events might differ from those of their family, friends or other collateral sources. In this case, you can record their accounts, followed by any collateral information available.

Previous psychiatric history

• Dates of illnesses, symptoms, diagnoses, treatments.
• Hospitalisations, including whether treatment was voluntary or compulsory.

Past medical/surgical history

• Dates of any serious medical illnesses.
• Dates of any surgical operations.
• Dates of any periods of hospitalisation.

Drug history and allergies

• All current medication.
Note psychotropic medications that patients have received previously, their dosage and duration, and whether or not they helped. It may be necessary to obtain this information from the patients' GP or hospital notes.

Family history

• Parents' and siblings' physical and mental health, their frequency of contact with, and the quality of their relationship with the patient.
• If a close relative is deceased, note the cause of death, the patient's age at the time of death and their reaction to that death (see Chapter 10).
• Ask about family history of psychiatric illness ('nervous breakdowns'), suicide or drug and/or alcohol abuse, forensic encounters and medical illnesses.

Personal history

• **Early life and development:** Include details of the pregnancy and birth (especially complications), any serious illnesses, bereavements, emotional, physical or sexual abuse, separations in childhood or developmental delays. Describe the childhood home environment (atmosphere and any deprivation). Note religious background and current religious beliefs/practices.
• **Educational history:** Include details of school, academic achievements, relationships with peers (did they have any friends?) and conduct (whether suspended, excluded or expelled). Bullying and school refusal or truancy should be explored.
• **Occupational history:** List job titles and duration, reasons for change; note work satisfaction and relationships with colleagues. The longest duration of continuous employment is a good indicator of premorbid functioning.
• **Relationship history:** Document details of relationships and marriages (duration, gender of partner, children, relationship quality, abuse); sexual difficulties; in the case of women, menstrual pattern, contraception, history of pregnancies. Those who are in a long-term relationship should be asked about the support they receive from their partner and the quality of the relationship – e.g. whether there is good communication, aggression (physical or verbal), jealousy or infidelity.

Substance use

• Alcohol, drug (prescribed and recreational) and tobacco consumption.

Forensic history

• Any arrests, whether they resulted in conviction and whether they were for violent offences.
• Any periods of imprisonment, for which offences and the length of time served.

Social history

• Describe current accommodation, occupation, financial situation and daily activities.

Premorbid personality

• A description of the patient's character and attitudes before they became unwell (e.g. character, social relations). You could ask:
  • How would you describe yourself before you became unwell?
  • How would your friends describe you?
  • What do you enjoy doing?
  • How do you usually cope when things go wrong?

2 The Mental State Examination

An example mental state

Appearance and behaviour: Mr Smith was a thin gentleman, appropriately dressed in casual clothes, with no evidence of poor personal hygiene or abnormal movements; he was not objectively hallucinating. He was polite, appropriate, maintained good eye contact and, although it was initially difficult to establish a rapport, this improved throughout the interview.
Speech: Normal in tone, rate and volume. Relevant and coherent, with no evidence of formal thought disorder.
Mood: Subjectively 'fine'; objectively euthymic.
Affect: Suspicious at times, particularly when discussing treatment; reactive.

Thoughts: Persecutory delusions and delusions of reference elicited (see 'History of the present illness', Chapter 1). Could not 'rule out' retaliating against neighbour, but no current thoughts, plans or intent to harm neighbour, self or anyone else. No evidence of depressive cognitions or anxiety symptoms. No suicidal ideation.
Perception: No abnormality detected.
Cognition: Alert, orientated to time, place and person. No impairment of concentration or memory noted during interview.
Insight: Patient feels stressed; he is aware that others think he has a psychotic illness but he disagrees with this. He does not want to receive any treatment and does not think he needs to be in hospital. He would be willing to see a counsellor for stress.

Appearance and behaviour

Here you should note:
• Their general health, build, posture, unusual tattoos or clothing, piercings, injection sites, lacerations (especially on the forearm).
• Whether they have good personal hygiene?
• Whether they are tidily dressed/well-kempt or unkempt?
• Their manner, rapport, eye contact, degree of cooperation, facial expression, whether responding to hallucinations.
• Motor activity may be excessive (psychomotor agitation) or decreased (psychomotor retardation).
• Abnormal movements may be antipsychotic side effects such as
  • tremor
  • bradykinesia: slowness of movement
  • akathisia: restlessness
  • tardive dyskinesia: usually affects the mouth, lips and tongue (e.g. rolling the tongue or licking the lips)
  • dystonia: muscular spasm causing abnormal face and body movement or posture.
• Other abnormal movements include:
  • tics
  • chorea
  • stereotypy: repetitive, purposeless movement (e.g. rocking in people with severe learning disability)
  • mannerisms: goal-directed, understandable movements (e.g. saluting)
  • gait abnormalities.

Speech

Describe tone (variation in pitch), rate (speed) and volume (quantity). In pressure of speech, rate and volume are increased and speech may be uninterruptible. In depression, tone, rate and volume are often decreased.
• 'Normal' speech can be described as 'spontaneous, logical, relevant and coherent'.

• 'Circumstantial' speech takes a long time to get to the point.
• Perseveration (repeating words or topics) is a sign of frontal lobe impairment.
• Neologisms (made up words e.g. 'headshoe' to mean 'hat') can occur in schizophrenia.

Thought form

• Normal speech consists of a series of phrases/statements connected by their meanings:
I am reading this book ⇒ because I want to pass my exam.
• In flight of ideas there is an abnormal connection between statements based on a rhyme or pun rather than meaning:
I read this book ⇒ because it was red and blue ⇒ I feel blue.
• In 'loosening of associations' there is no discernible link between statements:
I am reading ⇒ climate change ⇒ where's the piano?
• If you think a patient has abnormal thought form, record some examples of what they say.
• In thought block, the patient's subjective experience of thought is abnormal (thoughts disappear: 'my mind goes blank').

Mood and affect

• **Mood** is the underlying emotion; report subjective mood (in patient's own words) and objective mood (described as dysthymic (low), euthymic (normal) or hyperthymic (elated)).
• **Affect** is the observed (and often more transient) external manifestation of emotion. Mood has been compared to climate and affect to weather. An abnormal affect may be described as:
  • blunted/unreactive (lacking normal emotional responses – e.g. negative symptoms of schizophrenia)
  • labile (excessively changeable)
  • irritable (which may occur in mania, depression)
  • perplexed

Psychiatry at a Glance, Sixth Edition. Cornelius Katona, Claudia Cooper, Mary Robertson. © 2016 John Wiley & Sons, Ltd. Published 2016 by John Wiley & Sons, Ltd.
Companion website: www.ataglanceseries.com/psychiatry

- suspicious; or
  - incongruous (grossly out of tune with subjects being discussed – e.g. laughing about bereavement).
- Where no abnormality is detected, affect is described as reactive (appropriate response to emotional cues).

Disorders of thought content

Record:
- Negative (depressed) cognitions (e.g. guilt, hopelessness).
  - Ruminations (persistent, disabling preoccupations) that may occur in depression or anxiety (e.g. worrying about redundancy, illness or death).
  - Obsessions (Chapter 12) and phobias (Chapter 11).
  - Depersonalisation or derealisation: these often occur with anxiety; they are not psychotic phenomena.
  - Depersonalisation – feeling detached, unreal, watching oneself from the outside: 'as if cut off by a pane of glass'.
  - Derealisation – the world or people in it seeming lifeless: 'as if the world is made out of cardboard'.
- Abnormal beliefs. These are:
  - overvalued ideas: acceptable and comprehensible but pursued by the patient beyond the bounds of reason and to an extent that causes distress to them or others (e.g. an intense, non-delusional feeling of responsibility for a bereavement)
  - ideas of reference: thoughts that other people are looking at or talking about them, not held with delusional intensity
  - delusions: fixed, false, firmly held beliefs, out of keeping with the patient's culture and unaltered by contrary evidence.

Figure 2.1 Types of delusion

Delusion type:	Content	How to ask
Persecutory	Someone or something is interfering with the person in a malicious/destructive way	Do you worry that people are against you or trying to harm you?
Grandiose	Being famous, having supernatural power or enormous wealth	Do you have any exceptional abilities or talents?
Of reference	Actions of other people, events, media etc. are referring to the person or communicating a message	Have you heard people talking about you? Have you heard things on the TV or radio you think are about you?
Thought insertion/ withdrawal/ broadcast	Thoughts can be controlled by an outside influence: inserted, withdrawn or broadcast to others	Do you feel your thoughts are being interfered with or controlled? Are they known to others, e.g. through telepathy?
Passivity	Actions, feelings or impulses can be controlled or interfered with by outside influence	Do you feel another person can control what you do directly, as if they were pulling strings of a puppet?

- Ask about suicidal or homicidal ideation, plans and intent:

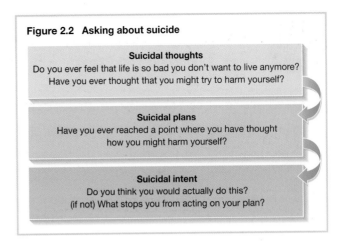

Figure 2.2 Asking about suicide

Suicidal thoughts
Do you ever feel that life is so bad you don't want to live anymore?
Have you ever thought that you might try to harm yourself?

Suicidal plans
Have you ever reached a point where you have thought how you might harm yourself?

Suicidal intent
Do you think you would actually do this?
(if not) What stops you from acting on your plan?

Perception

- Ask 'Have you seen or heard things that other people can't see or hear? Can you tell me more about that?'
- *Illusions* are misinterpretations of normal perceptions (e.g. interpreting a curtain cord as a snake). They can occur in healthy people.
- *Hallucinations* are perceptions, in the absence of an external stimulus, that are experienced as true and as coming from the outside world. They can occur in any sensory modality, although auditory and visual are the most common. Some auditory hallucinations occur in normal individuals when falling asleep (hypnagogic) or on waking (hypnopompic).
- *Pseudohallucinations* are internal perceptions with preserved insight (e.g. 'A voice inside my head tells me I'm no good.')

Cognition

Note at least the level of consciousness, memory, orientation, attention and concentration. More formal testing is needed for those who may have cognitive impairment and everyone aged 65 and over. This may involve completing a Mini-Mental State Examination (MMSE) with additional tests of frontal lobe function.

You should test:
- memory (e.g. repeating a list of three or more objects or an address – immediately and after 5 minutes)
- orientation in time (day, date, time), place, person (e.g. knowing their name, age and identity of relatives)
- attention and concentration (e.g. counting backwards)
- dyspraxia (e.g. drawing intersecting pentagons)
- receptive dysphasia (following a command)
- expressive dysphasia (naming objects)
- executive (frontal lobe) functioning tests such as:
  - approximation (e.g. height of a local landmark)
  - abstract reasoning (e.g. finding the next number or shape in a sequence)
  - verbal fluency (can they think of >15 words beginning with each of the letters F, A or S in a minute?)
  - proverb interpretation.

Insight

- The patient's understanding of their condition and its cause as well as their willingness to accept treatment.

3 Diagnosis and Classification in Psychiatry

Figure 3.1 ICD-10 and DSM-IV-TR diagnosis and classification

ICD-10	DSM-5	Main differences
F00–09 Organic disorders	Neurocognitive disorders	ICD-10 lists dementia subtypes (Alzheimer's, vascular) separately and MCI as a single category. DSM-5 distinguishes mild and major cognitive disorder for each subtype (so likely underlying pathology in MCI (e.g. Alzheimer type) specified in DSM-5
F10–19 Result of substance use	Substance-related and addictive disorders	ICD-10 separates *harmful use* and *dependence*, DSM-5 includes both as 'use disorder'. ICD-10 includes amnestic disorder (Chapter 18) here, DSM-5 as a neurocognitive disorder. DSM 5 includes gambling disorder here
F20–29 Psychotic disorders	Schizophrenia spectrum and other psychotic disorders	Schizophrenia requires 1 month of symptoms in ICD-10, 6 months in DSM-5. ICD-10 lists schizophrenia subtypes (e.g. paranoid, hebephrenic), DSM-5 doesn't. ICD-10 lists induced (shared) delusional disorders separately, in DSM-5 this is under delusional disorders; ICD-10 includes schizotypal disorder, in DSM-5 this is a personality disorder
F30–39 Mood (affective) disorders	Bipolar and related disorders	DSM-5 uses terms bipolar I disorder where ≥1 manic episode, bipolar II disorder where hypomanic but not manic episodes, ICD-10 does not
	Depressive disorders	ICD-10 requires 2/3 core symptoms for depression diagnosis (low mood/loss of enjoyment/low energy), DSM-5 one of low mood/loss of enjoyment. DSM-5 lists disruptive mood dysregulation disorder (explosive angry outbursts diagnosed < age 18, no ICD-10 equivalent) and premenstrual dysphoric disorder (physical disorder in ICD-10)
F40–49 Neurotic, stress-related and somatoform disorders	Anxiety disorders: • Obsessive-compulsive disorders • Trauma- and stressor-related disorders • Dissociative disorders • Somatic symptom and related disorders	DSM-5 specifies a duration of ≥6 months for phobias including agoraphobia, ICD-10 gives no minimum duration; DSM-5 lists some diagnoses here that ICD-10 includes as childhood disorders, e.g. in DSM-5 separation anxiety disorder and selective mutism can be diagnosed at any age. DSM-5 lists hoarding disorder (not in ICD-10); trichotillomania (hair-pulling disorder) (habit/impulse disorder in ICD-10) and body dysmorphic disorder (under hypochondriacal disorder in ICD-10) within obsessive compulsive disorders ICD-10 requires post traumatic stress disorder (PTSD) onset is within 6 months of stressor, in DSM-5 it is within 1 month
F50–59 Behavioural syndromes associated with physiological and physical factors	Feeding and eating disorders	ICD-10 requires amenorrhea for anorexia nervosa diagnosis, DSM-5 doesn't; in addition to anorexia and bulimia nervosas, DSM-5 includes *avoidant/restrictive food intake disorder and binge-eating disorder;* in ICD-10 *atypical anorexia and bulimia nervosas* and *overeating associated with psychological disturbance* are similar
	Sleep–wake disorders	
	Sexual dysfunctions	
F60–69 Personality, habit and impulse disorders, disorders of sexual preference and gender identity disorders	Personality disorders	DSM-5 lists antisocial personality disorder as a conduct disorder, ICD-10 includes dissocial personality disorder with other personality disorders. DSM-5 narcissistic personality disorder has no equivalent in ICD-10. ICD-10 includes *gender identity disorders*; DSM-5 introduced term *gender dysphoria* emphasizing 'gender incongruence' rather than cross-gender identification per se
	Paraphilic disorders	
	Disruptive, impulse-control and conduct disorders	
	Gender dysphoria	
F70–79 Mental retardation	Neurodevelopmental disorders: • Intellectual disability – communication, – autistic spectrum – motor (including tic) disorders	DSM-5 uses the term autistic spectrum disorder (ASD) to encompass autism, Asperger's syndrome and childhood disintegrative disorder, but ICD-10 lists these disorders separately. ASD has been the term used clinically in recent years and this reflects the more recent release of DSM-5
F80–89 Disorders of psychological development		
F90–98 Behavioural and emotional disorders, onset: childhood and adolescence		DSM-5 includes these diagnoses in other chapters – with adult emotional/ behavioural disorders and tic disorders with neurodevelopmental disorders

History

• Before the 1950s, diagnoses were unreliable and had meanings that varied across the world. In the 1960–1970s 'antipsychiatrists', including R. D. Laing and Thomas Szasz, suggested that psychiatric diagnoses should be abandoned, together with the concept of mental illness.

• The International Classification of Diseases (ICD) is a system developed by the World Health Organization (WHO) aimed at improving diagnosis and classification of disorders. The mental health section is currently in its tenth edition (ICD-10). Look online at some of the diagnostic criteria (http://apps.who.int/classifications/apps/icd/icd10online/). ICD 11 is scheduled for publication in 2017.

Psychiatry at a Glance, Sixth Edition. Cornelius Katona, Claudia Cooper, Mary Robertson. © 2016 John Wiley & Sons, Ltd. Published 2016 by John Wiley & Sons, Ltd.
Companion website: www.ataglanceseries.com/psychiatry

• The American Psychiatric Association developed its own classificatory system, the Diagnostic and Statistical Manual of Mental Disorders (DSM); the current classification, DSM 5 was released in May 2013.

• ICD-10 and DSM-5 are broadly similar. Figure 3.1 shows the main differences.

The concept of mental illness

• In medicine, a distinction is made between *disease* (objective physical pathology and known aetiology) and *illness* (subjective distress). Psychiatric conditions without known organic cause, such as depression, are described as illnesses or disorders not *diseases* since in many there is no demonstrable pathology. New techniques (e.g. neuroimaging) may identify definable psychiatric diseases.

• The concept of mental *illness* is useful in defining a level of subjective distress greater in severity or duration than occurs in normal human experience. The legislation in many countries requires psychiatrists to diagnose defined 'mental illness' when certifying the need for compulsory hospital treatment and in forensic (legal) psychiatry.

• Diagnostic criteria set thresholds to define the level of symptoms that constitute mental illness. These thresholds can be controversial. For example, compared to DSM-IV, DSM-5 criteria for ADHD are more inclusive – requiring symptoms before age 12 rather than age 7. In the USA, 20% of boys aged between 14 and 17 have been diagnosed with ADHD and 2/3 take medication. Critics claim this as the medicalization of childhood, proponents that it is right that those who may benefit from treatment receive it.

• Decisions about what constitutes mental illness change over time, influenced by:

1 Latest research findings e.g. gambling disorder is newly classified in DSM-5 among substance abuse/addictions as it has been found to have more in common with these disorders than with impulse control disorders where classified in DSM-IV.

2 Sociopolitical thinking: homosexuality was removed from the DSM in the 1970s. DSM-IV, gender identity disorder was changed to gender dysphoria in DSM-5 because 'gender incongruence' rather than cross-gender identification per se is considered a disorder.

Aims of classification in psychiatry

• To identify groups of patients who are similar in their clinical features, course of disease, outcome and response to treatment, aiding individual clinical management.

• To provide a common language for communication between patients, professionals and researchers.

• To improve the **reliability** (reproducibility among different settings) and **validity** (correctness) of diagnoses. Validity is more difficult to confirm but attempts have been made, including the examination of consistency of symptom patterns and demonstration of consistent treatment responses, long-term prognoses, genetic and biological correlates.

Categorical versus Dimensional

• ICD-10 and DSM-5 are **categorical systems**. They describe a group of discrete conditions. They give **operational definitions** specifying inclusion and exclusion criteria. These state which symptoms must be present for each diagnosis to be made (often quantifying their number and requiring a minimum duration).

• **Dimensional systems** use a continuum rather than categories and have been used mainly to classify personality. For example, Hans Eysenck proposed three dimensions of personality: introversion/extroversion, neuroticism (mental distress in which ability to distinguish between symptoms originating from patient's own mind and external reality is retained; includes most depressive and anxiety disorders) and psychoticism (severe mental disturbance characterised by a loss of contact with external reality). DSM-5 includes a suggested model for defining personality disorders that allows dimensional assessment of traits in its section for further study, although the main manual still defines personality disorders categorically.

Comorbidity

• Psychiatric diagnoses are made in ICD-10 (and to a lesser extent in DSM-5) using a diagnostic hierarchy, which is often illustrated as a triangle.

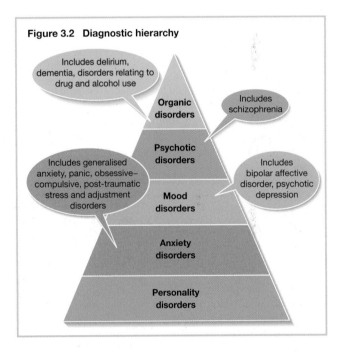

Figure 3.2 Diagnostic hierarchy

Includes delirium, dementia, disorders relating to drug and alcohol use

Includes schizophrenia

Includes generalised anxiety, panic, obsessive–compulsive, post-traumatic stress and adjustment disorders

Includes bipolar affective disorder, psychotic depression

Organic disorders

Psychotic disorders

Mood disorders

Anxiety disorders

Personality disorders

• Organic disorders are at the top of the triangle and take precedence when making diagnoses. For example, if a person with dementia is agitated and anxious, the anxiety would be classified as a neuropsychiatric symptom of the dementia rather than being diagnosed separately as anxiety disorder.

• Similarly, a person who met criteria for both a depressive episode and generalised anxiety disorder would be diagnosed with depression alone.

• Comorbidity (co-occurrence of two psychiatric disorders) is allowed in either system if a person is experiencing symptoms not explained by one diagnosis alone. For example, a person with an emotionally unstable personality disorder may be diagnosed with depression.

4 Risk Assessment and Management in Psychiatry

Figure 4.1 Balancing risks and patients' rights

Reduce risks to patients and potential victims

Respect patients' autonomy

Consider patients' right to mental health treatment

Management as unrestricting and unstigmatising as possible

KEY PRINCIPLES

Clinicians need to balance the need to reduce risk as far as possible with the duty to respect patients' rights and freedom; risk cannot be eliminated completely. This continuing process is called risk assessment and management.

Risk assessment

- All psychiatric patients should have a risk assessment to assess the level of risk they pose to themselves and to others (specific named people or risk of indiscriminate violence).
- This needs to be reviewed regularly since degree of risk is sensitive to changing circumstances and to a patient's changing mental state.
- Past behaviour is the best indicator of future behaviour and should be considered in addition to the current episode history and mental state.
- History from informants (e.g. family, hostel staff) and a review of case notes and other documentation are critical to ensure all important information is considered.
- Assess patients in as safe an environment as possible – assessment areas should have appropriate alarm facilities and easily available exit routes. Consider potential access to harmful agents (firearms, knives, other weapons, incendiary devices, objects that can be used as weapons). Where risk behaviour is anticipated, ensure that senior staff and appropriate security/support staff are present where possible.

Risk of self-harm

From the psychiatric interview and case notes, document:
- current suicidal thoughts, plans and intent;
- anything that prevents the patient acting on these thoughts (e.g. family, religion);
- previous episodes of deliberate self-harm (circumstances, method and management);
- factors predisposing to deliberate self-harm or actual suicide (see Chapter 7), which include:
  - a family history of suicide
  - social isolation
  - substance misuse

- any history of previous disengagement from statutory or voluntary support services, and whether the patient is now willing to engage with such services.

In the mental state examination, look for these risk factors:
- thoughts of hopelessness and worthlessness.
- command hallucinations inciting self-harm.

Risk of harm to others

From the psychiatric interview and case notes, document:
- acts or threats of violence (to whom directed, frequency, severity, methods used and most serious harm resulting);
- deliberate arson;
- sexually inappropriate behaviour;
- episodes of containment (compulsory detention, treatment in special hospital, secure unit, locked ward, prison or police station);
- extent of compliance with previous and current psychiatric treatment and aftercare; note past or current episodes of disengagement from psychiatric follow-up.

Document the following because they can increase risk:
- recent discontinuation of prescribed drugs;
- change in use of recreational drugs;
- alcohol or drug misuse (or any other disinhibiting factors);
- impulsive or unpredictable behaviour;
- recent stressful life events, changes in personal circumstances, lack or loss of social support, because these may indicate 'social restlessness' (frequent changes of relationships, work or domicile).

In the mental state examination, look for:
- expressed violent intentions or threats;
- irritability, disinhibition, suspiciousness;
- persecutory delusions (especially with specific person or people involved);
- delusions of control or passivity phenomena;
- command hallucinations.

Risk to children (those referred in their own right or whose parents have a mental illness) should be assessed. Both confidentiality (with regards the patient) and duty to the child must be considered carefully and, if in doubt, advice taken.

Risk of self-neglect and accidental harm

People with mental illness may lack the motivation (e.g. because of severe depression, chronic schizophrenia) or skills (dementia, learning disability) to care for themselves and/or to arrange access to necessary services (e.g. heating, lighting, housing and health care). This can result in serious health risks from:
- malnutrition (forgetting to eat, eating out-of-date food);
- failure to access health care or living in squalid conditions;
- falls owing to physical frailty or alcohol or drug intoxication;
- failure to take adequate safeguards against fire (cigarette-burned bedclothes indicate such a risk) or explosion (from leaving the gas on);

Psychiatry at a Glance, Sixth Edition. Cornelius Katona, Claudia Cooper, Mary Robertson. © 2016 John Wiley & Sons, Ltd. Published 2016 by John Wiley & Sons, Ltd.
Companion website: www.ataglanceseries.com/psychiatry

- wandering (leaving the house and being unable to find the way home, or going out at inappropriate times such as middle of night), poor road safety;
- accidentally taking too much or too little medication;
- vulnerability to crime through leaving the front door open, persistently losing door key or inviting strangers in.

Vulnerability to abuse

- Abuse is defined as a single or repeated act or lack of appropriate action occurring within any relationship where there is an expectation of trust and which causes harm or distress to a vulnerable (e.g. older or learning disabled) person. Abuse may be verbal, psychological, physical, financial, sexual or through neglect.
- People living in institutions may be at particular risk.
- Abuse also occurs in private homes and this may relate to high levels of stress in family carers. Carers are sometimes at the receiving end of verbal or physical abuse and this should also be enquired into.

Risks to vulnerable adults: how safe?

HOme safety (e.g. leaving gas on)
Wandering

Self neglect (e.g. poor self care)
Abuse, neglect, crime vulnerability
Falls
Eating (malnutrition)

Managing violence
Immediate management

- For community patients, consider whether admission is necessary, and, if so, whether this should be under the Mental Health Act (Chapters 40–42), possibly to a psychiatric intensive care unit (PICU) or secure unit.
- All staff working in psychiatry should be trained in 'breakaway' techniques for escaping from violent situations. Nursing staff in psychiatric units are trained in safe methods of control and restraint of patients, the first stage of which is always to try to manage the situation by 'talking down'.
- Medication can be used to treat any underlying psychiatric disorder and (in patients with high levels of arousal) for sedation or tranquilisation; usually benzodiazepines and/or antipsychotic medication are used (see Chapters 34 and 36).
- Very occasionally, it is necessary to manage violent and aggressive patients in seclusion for short periods of time to ensure the safety of staff and other patients.

Managing violence: be careful

Breakaway
Evaluate and talk down

Control and restraint
Assess need for medication to sedate and/or treat disorder
RE-evaluate setting (is higher level of security needed?)
FULly review care plan

Preventing future violence

- Level of monitoring should be specified for patients in the community and for those in hospital.
- Communication between agencies (particularly Health, Probation and Social Services) is crucial, especially for high-risk patients.
- Care plans and their implementation must be negotiated by all involved parties (including the patients themselves, their families and other informal carers) and fully documented.
- Document all incidents and new information that may suggest a change in risk. Even if a piece of information seems insignificant, it may not be when considered together with information from other sources or time points.

Preventing violence: warn

Write risk incidents in notes
Assess in a safe environment
Read documentation before you assess
Notify professionals involved of risks

Breaking confidentiality

- Patients have a right to expect that information about them will be held in confidence by their doctors.
- If professionals are aware of a specific threat to a named individual, they have a duty to ensure that the person concerned is informed.
- In very rare circumstances, disclosure of patients' information may be justified in the public interest, even if the patients withhold their consent (e.g. if disclosure may assist in the prevention, detection or prosecution of a serious crime).
- Professionals also have a responsibility to report significant abuse that may cause, or has caused, harm to children and vulnerable adults (people with dementia or learning disabilities, or others who cannot make decisions about their own welfare) to appropriate agencies (Social Services or, in very serious cases, the police).
- Seek senior advice if in any doubt about breaking confidentiality.

5 Suicide and Deliberate Self-harm

Figure 5.1 Key facts about suicide and deliberate self-harm

	Suicide	Deliberate self-harm (DSH)
Definition	Intentional self-inflicted death	Intentional non-fatal self-inflicted harm
Incidence	8/100 000 per year	2–3/1000 per year
Epidemiology	M > F ▲ Middle aged men (40–50)	F > M ▲ Younger women
Aetiology	• Availability of means • ▼ Social support • Life events • Mental illness: – depression – schizophrenia – substance misuse – emotionally unstable or antisocial personality disorder – eating disorder	
	• Chronic painful illnesses • Family history of suicide • ▼ Brain Derived Neurotrophic Factor at postmortem	• Unemployed, divorce • Socioeconomic deprivation

Suicide

Epidemiology

• There are about 8 suicides per 100 000 people per year in UK (1% of all deaths).

• UK suicide rates have fallen in the past decade with a small increase in the period 2010–2014, probably as a result of the global economic crisis.

• Suicides worldwide are more common in men than women; in the UK the highest suicide rates are in middle aged (aged 40–50) men, and around three-quarters of victims are men.

• The most frequently used methods vary between countries and by gender. In the USA, most deaths involve firearms; in the UK hanging is more common in men, hanging and self-poisoning in women. Other methods include jumping in front of a train or car and exsanguination; worldwide, pesticide ingestion is common. Firearms are more often used by male suicide victims.

Aetiology

The aetiology of any suicide is likely to be a complex interplay of factors, but the following are often important:

• **Mental illness**: Retrospective 'psychiatric autopsy' studies have suggested that a current psychiatric diagnosis can be made in almost all suicides. Recent UK statistics show:

  • Just under 20% of all mental health patient suicides were within three months of discharge from inpatient psychiatric care, 10% happened in current inpatients, 8% in those in contact with Crisis Resolution and home treatment teams (CR/HTT). Disorders frequently implicated include:

  – substance misuse – 56% had a history of alcohol or drug misuse;

  – schizophrenia – 16% had this diagnosis;

  – severe mental illness and substance misuse diagnoses – 15%;

  – personality disorder – the primary diagnosis in 8% of suicides, 71% of whom had comorbid depression or substance misuse;

  – depression – very commonly implicated, often comorbid with other disorders.

• Suicide rates are also particularly high in prisons because of high rates of mental illness, deprivation and stress.

Other risk factors include:

• Chronic painful illnesses.

• Availability of means: removing potential ligature points from inpatient wards, restrictive firearm legislation and reducing paracetamol and aspirin pack sizes have reduced suicide rates.

• Family history of suicide.

• Lack of social support or recent adverse life events (loss of job, bereavement, divorce or other loss of relationship).

Emile Durkheim's 'types' of suicide

Anomic suicide: reflects a society's disintegration and loss of common values. This is demonstrated by positive correlations between suicide rates and unemployment and homicide rates, and reductions in suicide in wartime and other moments of social unity in adversity – rates dropped in New York after the terrorist attack of September 2001.

Egoistic suicide: involves individuals' separation from otherwise cohesive social groups. Demonstrated by higher suicide rates following bereavement and moving house, in immigrants and people living alone, and the divorced or single, compared with people who are married (but social isolation is also frequently the consequence of major mental illnesses).

Altruistic suicide: for the good of society (e.g. Kamikaze pilots in the Second World War).

• At a biological level, expression of Brain Derived Neurotrophic Factor (BDNF) is reduced in the brains of people who have committed suicide.

• Countries where Finno-Ugrian (Finnish and Hungarian) ethnicities prevail show some of the highest suicide rates in Europe and worldwide, suggesting there may be genetic susceptibility factors (relating to heritable behavioural and personality traits, such as aggression, depression and impulsivity).

Suicide prevention strategies

• Detect and treat psychiatric disorders.

• Be alert to risk and respond appropriately to it. A large proportion of people who commit suicide have consulted their general practitioners (GPs) in the previous few weeks.

• Prescribe safely – e.g. prescribing of co-proxamol must take account of the fact that an overdose of relatively few tablets may be lethal, especially if consumed with alcohol.

• Give urgent care at appropriate level of patients with suicide intent – CR/HTT or hospitalization (consider detention under the Mental Health Act) if patients considered unsafe outside hospital even with intensive support.

• Provide careful management of deliberate self-harm (DSH) because there is a high risk of repetition including completed suicide (see next section).

• Act at the population level, tackling unemployment and reducing access to methods of self-harm.

DSH
Epidemiology and correlates

• DSH is a much (20–30 times) more common event than completed suicide, with an annual incidence of 2–3/1000 in the UK.

• DSH significantly increases the risk of completed suicide. A third of suicide victims have self-harmed at least once in the past.

• Most cases involve drug overdose or physical self-injury (e.g. cutting or stabbing).

• Unlike completed suicide, DSH is more frequent in women, the under-35s, lower social classes and the single or divorced.

• Like suicide, DSH is associated with psychiatric illness, particularly depression and personality disorder.

• In borderline personality disorder, repetitive self-harm (commonly superficial wrist cutting) may be carried out to relieve tension rather than because of a wish to die.

Assessment

• The immediate priority is medical stabilisation. Subsequent psychiatric assessment first involves establishing rapport with the patient and adopting a non-judgemental approach.

• DSH is often precipitated by undesirable life events. In most cases, its motive can be understood in terms of one or more of:
  • a desire to *interrupt* a sequence of events seen as inevitable and undesirable
  • a need for *attention*
  • an attempt to *communicate*
  • a true *wish to die*.

• The latter, although probably the single best indicator of high subsequent risk of suicide, is seldom unequivocal or stable.

Relevant interview topics include:
• identification of motive(s), acute and chronic problems and associated coping strategies;
• screening for current psychiatric illness;
• screening for indicators of high risk: leaving a suicide note, making a will, continued determination to die, marked feelings of hopelessness and an attempt carefully prepared with precautions taken to prevent discovery and high lethality risk, either objectively or as imagined by the patient;
• social history: risk is higher in older, male, unemployed or socially isolated individuals;
• history of self-harm; risk of repeated non-fatal DSH is highest in subjects of low social class, with antisocial or emotionally unstable personality disorder, no work and/or a criminal record, and in those who abuse substances.

Options for DSH management

> **Mediate**
>
> **M**edically stabilise
> **E**stablish rapport
> **D**iagnose and treat mental illness
> **I**atrogenic risk – prescribe safely
> **A**ssess likelihood of recurrence:
> **T**houghts might return – make a plan
> **E**valuate social problems

• The objectives of DSH management are to:
  • decrease risk of repetition and of completed suicide
  • initiate or continue treatment of any underlying psychiatric illness
  • address ongoing social difficulties.

• A good first step is to agree with patients what their problems are and what immediate interventions are both feasible and acceptable to them.

• Ensure that they know who they can turn to if suicidal intent returns (e.g. A & E). Inpatient admission is needed for a minority; compulsory admission may be indicated where a patient has active suicidal intent.

• Crisis Resolution Team referral may be necessary if suicidal ideation is present.

• Think about reducing access to means of suicide if possible – for example, by encouraging patients to dispose of unneeded tablets from the home, and by prescribing antidepressants of lower lethality (e.g. SSRIs rather than tricyclics) and in small batches.

• Consider psychological therapy and encouraging engagement in self-help and community social and support organisations. Dialectical behaviour therapy (see Chapter 33) can reduce repetitive self-harm in emotionally unstable personality disorder.

Outcome

• A fifth of people who self-harm repeat their act within a year.

• Risk of actual suicide within a year is 1–2%; this is 100 times higher than in the general population.

• Prior DSH (particularly in people with depression, bipolar disorder or schizophrenia) is the best predictor of future completed suicide.

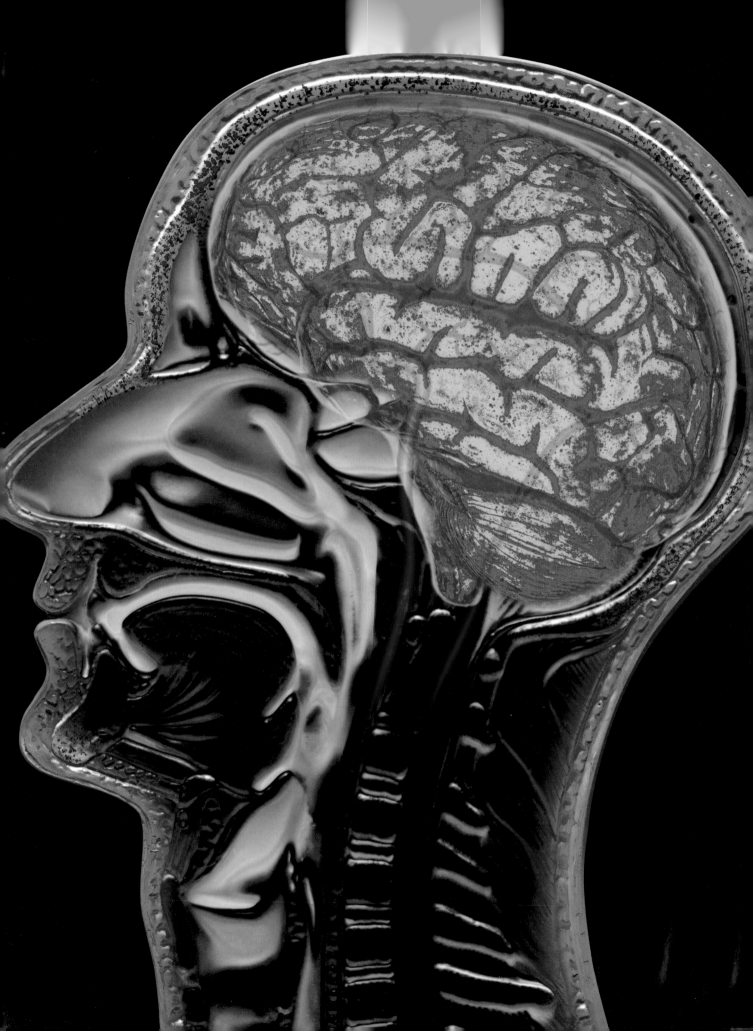

Mental Disorders

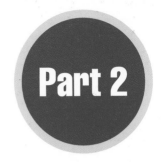

Part 2

Chapters

6 Psychosis: Symptoms and Aetiology

Figure 6.1 ICD-10: symptoms required for diagnosis of schizoprenia

One of these ...	How to ask
Delusions	
Persecutory delusions	Do you have any enemies? Do you feel that anyone is out to get you?
Delusions of reference	Do you ever see or hear things that you feel are giving a message that is specific to you?
Delusional perception (delusion arises from real perception, e.g. 'from bunch of flowers by road, I knew terrorists were after me')	
Thought insertion/withdrawal/broadcast (thoughts interfered with)	Are your thoughts being interfered with or controlled? Are they known to others, e.g. through telepathy?
Passivity (actions, feelings or impulses interfered with)	Can another person control what you do/ feel directly?
Somatic passivity (body controlled by others)	
Hallucinations	
Third-person auditory hallucinations (discussing/giving running commentary)	Do you hear people talking whom others can't hear? What do they say?
Or two of these...	
Any type of persistent hallucination (includes thought echo (hear own thoughts out loud) which is a Schneiderian first rank symptom)	Do you see/smell/taste things that others can't see/hear/taste
Neologisms (made-up words) or other forms of disorganised speech/ though disorder	Observed
'Negative' symptoms, e.g. apathy, poverty of speech, blunted or incongruous emotional responses	Observed

Schneider's first rank symptoms Schneider's second rank symptoms

Psychosis describes the misperception of thoughts and perceptions that arise from the patient's own mind/imagination as reality, and includes delusions and hallucinations. It is a symptom, not a diagnosis. About 3% of the general population has clinically significant psychosis. Psychotic disorders include: schizophrenia, delusional disorder, schizoaffective disorder, psychotic depression and bipolar affective disorder (Chapter 9).

Schizophrenia
History
• Emil Kraepelin (1893) divided psychotic disorders into *manic depression*, where normal function was regained between periods of relapse, and *dementia praecox*, characterised by irreversible deterioration of mental functions. The latter corresponds broadly to current concepts of schizophrenia.
• Bleuler coined the term, 'schizophrenia' in 1911.
• Kurt Schneider (1959) described **first and second rank symptoms of schizophrenia** (see Figure 6.1) – first rank symptoms are highly suggestive of schizophrenia but also occur in 8% of patients with bipolar affective disorder, while 20% of people with

chronic schizophrenia never show them. Current ICD-10 and DSM-5 classifications are strongly based on these.

Epidemiology
• The annual incidence of schizophrenia is 15–20/100 000, with a lifetime risk of 0.7%. Lifetime risk is greater in men (1.4:1). Peak incidence is in late teens or early adulthood.

Symptoms
These can be divided into:
• Positive symptoms:
  • delusions, most commonly persecutory or delusions of reference (see also Chapter 2)
  • hallucinations
  • formal thought disorder (disorganised speech) e.g. loosening of associations (Chapter 2), neologisms (new words, or words used in a special way).
• Negative symptoms:
  • poverty of speech, flat affect, poor motivation, social withdrawal and lack of concern for social conventions.
• Cognitive symptoms:
  • poor attention and memory.

Diagnosis

- Current diagnostic criteria are still broadly based on Schneider's First Rank Symptoms. The diagnosis should not be made in the presence of drug intoxication or withdrawal, overt brain disease or prominent affective symptoms.
  - **ICD-10** requires that certain symptoms (see Figure 6.1) are present for at least a month.
  - **DSM-5** requires at least two of the following, including one positive symptom (1–3 below) are present for at least six months:
    1. delusions
    2. hallucinations
    3. disorganized speech
    4. disorganized or catatonic behaviour
    5. negative symptoms.

Subtypes of schizophrenia

ICD-10 includes these subtypes. DSM-5 does not list subtypes because of their limited validity in predicting treatment response.

- *Paranoid* schizophrenia, the most common, in which delusions and auditory hallucinations are evident.
- *Catatonic* schizophrenia is uncommon (about 7% of cases). Psychomotor disturbances are prominent, often alternating between motor immobility (e.g. stupor) and excessive activity. Rigidity, posturing (e.g. waxy flexibility – maintaining strange postures), echolalia (copying speech) and echopraxia (copying behaviours) may occur.
- *Hebephrenic* schizophrenia: early onset and poor prognosis. Behaviour is irresponsible and unpredictable; mood inappropriate and affect incongruous, perhaps with giggling, mannerisms, and pranks; thought incoherence and fleeting delusions and hallucinations occur.
- *Residual schizophrenia:* there is a history of one of the types of schizophrenia described above, but in the current illness 'negative' and often cognitive symptoms predominate.
- *Simple schizophrenia:* uncommon; negative symptoms without preceding overt psychotic symptoms.

At risk of psychosis

- Acute psychotic illness may be preceded by a **prodromal** period during which patients exhibit symptoms such as anxiety, depression and ideas of reference (feelings of being watched).
- If a person is distressed, has a decline in social functioning and has transient psychotic symptoms, behaviour suggestive of possible psychosis or a first-degree relative with psychosis, they may be at risk of psychosis
- People at risk may be offered CBT and treatment of comorbid conditions, but not antipsychotic medication.

Aetiology

- **Genetics**: schizophrenia and affective psychoses are more prevalent in relatives of people with schizophrenia. The risk of developing schizophrenia is around 50% in someone who has a monozygotic twin with the disorder, 15% if a dizygotic twin is affected. Offspring of people with schizophrenia brought up in adopted families still have an increased (about 12%) chance of developing it. A number of genes affecting brain development probably contribute to this increased susceptibility. Advanced paternal age has been identified as a risk factor, probably owing to increased risk of chromosomal aberrations.
- *Neurodevelopmental hypothesis:* factors that interfere with early brain development lead to an increased risk of schizophrenia in adulthood. Evidence for this includes increased rates of schizophrenia associated with:
  - winter births (foetus more likely to be exposed to influenza);
  - obstetric complications, low birth weight and perinatal injuries;
  - developmental delay and poor academic performance ;
  - 'soft' neurological signs (e.g. abnormal movements, mixed-handedness);
  - temporal lobe epilepsy;
  - smoking cannabis in adolescence;
  - severe childhood bullying or physical abuse.

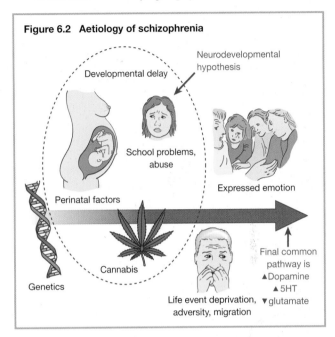

Figure 6.2 Aetiology of schizophrenia

The neurodevelopmental hypothesis is also supported by findings of increased ventricular size and small amounts of grey matter loss from CT/MRI studies of people with schizophrenia.

- **Social factors:** Schizophrenia is also associated with socioeconomic deprivation, urbanity and an excess of *life events* in the 3 weeks before the onset of acute symptoms. In the UK, the incidence of all psychoses is higher in African Caribbeans and Black Africans than the White British population (see Chapter 23). People with schizophrenia living in families with high expressed emotion (relatives over-involved or making hostile or excessive critical comments) are more likely to relapse.
- *Neurochemical changes:* The way in which genetic, neurodevelopmental and social factors result in schizophrenia in vulnerable individuals is not clearly understood, but the final common pathway appears to involve dopamine excess or overactivity in mesolimbic dopaminergic pathways (stimulant drugs such as amphetamines release dopamine and lead to psychosis; antipsychotics, which block dopamine receptors, treat psychosis successfully). Raised serotonin and decreased glutamate activity have also been implicated.

Other psychoses

- **Schizoaffective disorder** - affective and schizophrenic symptoms occur together and with equal prominence
- **Delusional disorder** - a fixed delusion or delusional system (associated delusions) with other areas of thinking and functioning well preserved.
- **Brief psychotic episodes** - last less time than required for schizophrenia diagnosis (1 month in ICD, 6 months in DSM).

7 Schizophrenia: Management and Prognosis

Figure 7.1 Management of psychosis

Management of psychosis

Treat acute episode	Reduce risk of relapse	Promote long-term recovery
Intervene early: prompt treatment associated with better outcome		
ANTIPSYCHOTICS • Lowest effective dose • Usually oral (occasionally depot, IM) • Monitor side effects • Adherence	Maintenance treatment reduced relapse rate if continued > 1–2 years after acute episode	• Maintenance treatment
PSYCHOLOGICAL THERAPY • Self-help to come to terms with symptoms/illness	Family therapy to reduce expressed emotion	• CBT to help manage residual symptoms • Art therapy to help negative symptoms
SOCIAL SUPPORT • Focus on engagement, hope, reduce stigma	Support to reduce substance misuse	• Support employment and study • Appropriate accommodation

This chapter mainly concerns the treatment of schizophrenia, the most common non-affective psychosis. The principles are relevant to all psychoses.

• People with schizophrenia and other psychotic disorders face considerable stigma, and public understanding of the disorder is limited. Care should be given with sensitivity, hope and optimism. Engagement is critical for the patient's subsequent adherence and prognosis.

• Early detection and intervention is important.

• The longer the period between symptom onset and effective treatment (**Duration of Untreated Psychosis**), the worse the average outcome.

• The first few years after onset can be particularly distressing with a high risk of suicide.

• Therefore, in many developed countries, specialist **Early Intervention in Psychosis** teams support people in the first few years of their illness.

• People with psychosis are treated in the community rather than in hospital wherever possible, although admission may be necessary if the risks of serious neglect, suicide/deliberate self-harm or harm to others are high. If the patient refuses treatment, formal admission under the Mental Health Act may be required.

• After the first acute episode, the treatment focus shifts to promoting long-term recovery. People with schizophrenia face problems of social exclusion and barriers to returning to work or study.

• Including carers and family in care plans is important, unless this is against the patient's wishes.

Medication

• Antipsychotics are effective in treating 'positive symptoms' in the acute episode (e.g. hallucinations, delusions, passivity phenomena) and in preventing relapses.

• Typical (conventional) and atypical (second-generation) antipsychotics are equally effective in the treatment of positive symptoms but have different side-effect profiles. 'Atypical' antipsychotics cause fewer motor side effects, but some are associated with weight gain and diabetes (see Chapter 34 for more about side effects and their treatment). The choice of antipsychotic should be made together with the patient, after explaining the relative side-effect profiles.

• After baseline investigations (see Chapter 34), treatment should be with the lowest dose that effectively controls symptoms to minimise side effects because these are associated with poor treatment adherence. The use of two antipsychotics concurrently should be avoided.

• Newly diagnosed patients should be offered oral medication. Liquid and orodispersible tablet formulations can be useful. Depot preparations may be used if this is the patient's preference or avoiding covert non-adherence is a clinical priority. Patients who are agitated, overactive or violent may require sedation (with antipsychotics or benzodiazepines). This may need to be by intra-muscular injection.

• The medication should be taken at optimal dose for 4–6 weeks before deciding if it is effective. Patients should be regularly reviewed, noting the effectiveness of treatment, side effects, adherence and physical health. As weight gain, cardiac arrhythmias and diabetes may also be problematic during treatment

Psychiatry at a Glance, Sixth Edition. Cornelius Katona, Claudia Cooper, Mary Robertson. © 2016 John Wiley & Sons, Ltd. Published 2016 by John Wiley & Sons, Ltd.
Companion website: www.ataglanceseries.com/psychiatry

with atypical antipsychotic drugs, patients require regular monitoring of weight, lipid and glucose profiles, and ECGs.

• Only clozapine has been shown to be effective in the treatment of psychosis that does not respond to treatment with other antipsychotic drugs. It is reserved for patients who do not respond to two other drugs. Blood monitoring is required because of potentially dangerous side effects (see Chapter 34).

• There is a high risk of relapse if antipsychotic medication is stopped within one to two years of an acute psychotic episode. Many clinicians advise continuing treatment for five years after an acute episode.

• People with schizophrenia can develop depression requiring treatment.

Psychological treatment

• NICE guidelines (2014) state that all people with schizophrenia should be offered individual **cognitive behavioural therapy** (CBT), and their families should be offered family interventions.

• CBT can help patients cope with persistent delusions and hallucinations. The aim is to alleviate distress and disability, and not necessarily to eliminate symptoms. Therapy might include encouraging a patient to:

   • learn to challenge or think differently about a voice (auditory hallucination) and to be less frightened of it;
   • develop strategies to cope with hearing voices – such as using distraction (e.g. listening to music) or telling the voices to go away;
   • challenge delusional beliefs and think of other possible explanations.

• Psychological support is important for all people with schizophrenia and their families. **Family therapy** helps families reduce their excessive expressed emotion (see Chapter 6), and there is good evidence that it is effective in preventing relapses.

• **Art therapies** can be particularly helpful for negative symptoms.

• **Self-help** groups and forums (e.g. Hearing Voices groups) enable people with psychosis to share experiences and ways to cope with symptoms.

Social support

• Helping people to return to work or study is crucial in maintaining their self-esteem and quality of life. Supported employment programmes should be offered. Where a return to work or study is not possible, day centres can provide daytime structure.

• Appropriate accommodation is important. People with residual symptoms (e.g. negative or cognitive symptoms) may not be able to live independently. Inpatient and community rehabilitation services aim to maximise independence (e.g. by teaching daily living skills). A range of supported living arrangements, from 24-hour staffed hostels to independent housing with support workers who visit once a week, are available depending on need.

Prognosis

• Seventy per cent of people experiencing a first psychotic episode will be well within a year, but 80% have a further episode within five years.

• Three-quarters of patients will discontinue their initial medication within the first 18 months, and those who do may be five times more likely to relapse over this period. In addition to taking medication, avoiding illicit drug use (in particular, cannabis) and excessive stress will reduce the risk of relapse.

• Only about 40% of people with schizophrenia will be in paid employment a year after their first episode; for those with multiple episodes, employment rates are even lower.

• Better prognosis is encountered in the developing world; this may be because of differences in social structure, greater family support or less stigma.

• Here are some factors associated with a good prognosis:

Good prognostic factors

Female
In relationship, good social support
No negative symptoms
a**D**heres to medication
Intelligence (more educated)
No stress
Good premorbid personality

Paranoid subtype
Late onset
Acute onset
No substance misuse
Scan (CT/MRI brain) normal

• The lifetime suicide risk is 10%. Suicide risk is higher:
   • in young men,
   • in the first few years of illness,
   • when there are persistent hallucinations or delusions,
   • when there is a history of illicit drug use,
   • when there have been previous suicide attempts.

8 Depression

Definitions and classification

- The most common symptom of depressive illness is a pervasive lowering of mood, although this is not essential for a diagnosis to be made. ICD-10 identifies three core symptoms, at least two of which should be present every day for at least two weeks:
  - low mood
  - anhedonia (loss of enjoyment in formerly pleasurable activities)
  - decreased energy (or increased fatiguability).
- Other symptoms include:
  - reduced concentration and attention
  - reduced self-esteem and self-confidence
  - ideas of guilt and worthlessness
  - feelings of hopelessness regarding the future
  - thoughts of self-harm
  - decreased sleep and/or appetite.
- The severity of the episode (mild, moderate, severe) depends on:
  - the number of symptoms present
  - the severity of symptoms
  - the degree of associated distress
  - interference with daily activities.
- Depression associated with psychotic features is always classified as severe.
- DSM-5 diagnostic criteria for major depressive disorder (its term for clinical depression) are similar, but one core symptom, either low mood or loss of enjoyment, is required.
- Mood disorders with recurrent episodes are described as unipolar if they include only depressive episodes, or bipolar if there is a history of at least one manic or hypomanic episode. Many unipolar depressed patients with a bipolar family history, very early onset and marked agitation subsequently meet criteria for bipolar disorder.

Clinical features

- Thought content often includes negative, pessimistic thoughts about:

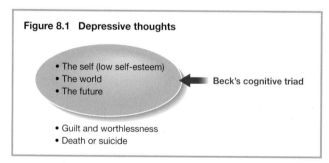

Figure 8.1 Depressive thoughts

- The self (low self-esteem)
- The world
- The future

Beck's cognitive triad

- Guilt and worthlessness
- Death or suicide

- Biological symptoms (e.g. reduced sleep, appetite and libido) may be particularly prominent in older people, who less often complain of disturbed mood. There is often a sleep pattern of early waking (more than two hours before usual) and maximal lowering of mood in the morning (diurnal variation). Poor appetite is often associated with weight loss; in severe cases, food and fluids may be refused.
- Motor activity is often altered, with psychomotor agitation, retardation (of speech and/or movement), or both.
- Cognition may be impaired, with reduced attention, concentration and decisiveness.
- Depressive symptoms can be masked by severe anxiety, alcohol, hypochondriacal preoccupations or irritability.
- Anhedonia is usually accompanied by loss of motivation and emotional reactivity.
- Psychotic features may occur and are usually mood-congruent. Delusions are usually nihilistic (e.g. a belief that one is dead, has lost all one's assets or one's body is rotting), delusional or hypochondriacal, concerning illness or death. Where hallucinations occur they are usually auditory, in the second person and accusing, condemning or urging the individual to commit suicide.
- Atypical depression is characterised by initial anxiety-related insomnia, subsequent oversleeping, increased appetite and a relatively bright, reactive mood. It is more common in adolescence.
- Depression is often also comorbid with anxiety disorders, eating disorders, personality disorders and substance misuse.

Differential diagnosis

- Normal sadness, particularly in the context of bereavement (Chapter 10) or severe physical illness. The diagnosis depends on finding a pattern of characteristic features and on the degree and duration of associated disability. Predominant negative, guilty or suicidal thoughts support a diagnosis of depression, but such symptoms may be difficult to elicit if depression is severe.
- Psychotic depression should be differentiated from schizophrenia (Chapter 6) on the basis of thought content (mood-congruent psychotic features) and the temporal sequence in which the symptoms developed.
- Depressive retardation may be difficult to distinguish from the flat (unreactive) affect of chronic schizophrenia (Chapter 6).
- Alcohol or drug withdrawal may mimic depression.

Epidemiology

- The lifetime risk of depression is about 10–20%, with rates almost doubled in women.
- First onset is typically in the third decade (earlier for bipolar disorder).
- Depression is strongly associated with socioeconomic deprivation.

Aetiology

- A genetic contribution is evident in both twin and adoption studies but less markedly for unipolar than bipolar depression. Current theories implicate gene-environment interactions – i.e. a genetic predisposition to depression if exposed to adverse life events.

- Monoamine neurotransmitter availability (particularly noradrenaline and serotonin) in the synaptic cleft is reduced in depressed patients, and antidepressants increase monoamine availability. It is now thought that this results in secondary neuroplastic changes that bring about the antidepressant effect. One suggested mechanism is that the greater monoamine availability leads to increased production of Brain Derived Neurotrophic Factor (BDNF) that promotes neurogenesis.

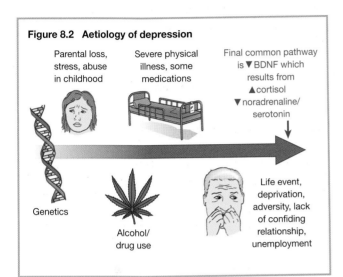

Figure 8.2 Aetiology of depression

Parental loss, stress, abuse in childhood

Severe physical illness, some medications

Final common pathway is ▼ BDNF which results from ▲ cortisol ▼ noradrenaline/ serotonin

Genetics

Alcohol/ drug use

Life event, deprivation, adversity, lack of confiding relationship, unemployment

- Hypercortisolaemia has been reported in severe depression, while in atypical depression hypocortisolaemia has been reported.
- The limbic system and related areas such as the prefrontal cortex regulate emotion, reward and executive function, and dysfunctional changes have been implicated in depression. Deep brain stimulation of the subgenual cingulate cortex or the nucleus accumbens has an antidepressant effect.
- Psychosocial factors implicated are recent adverse life events (e.g. bereavement or deteriorating physical health) and adverse current social circumstances, especially unemployment and lack of a confiding relationship. Parental loss and major childhood stress or abuse appear to increase vulnerability to depression in adulthood. Stress leads to increased cortisol levels, which may cause depressed mood through decreasing expression of BDNF.
- Cytokines are also important modulators of mood. Interleukin 1 (IL-1) produces 'sickness behaviour' in rodents. A third of those treated with recombinant interferons develop depression.
- Several physical illnesses (most endocrine disorders, many cancers, some viral infections) and some medications (including steroids, isotretinoin (for acne)) are specifically associated with depression.
- Women are particularly vulnerable to episodes of depression in the weeks following childbirth.

Management

- Most depressive illnesses can be managed in primary care, although many are undetected. Psychiatric referral is indicated if suicide risk is high or if the depression is severe, unresponsive to initial treatment, bipolar or recurrent.
- Depressed patients often present with other conditions.
- Always assess risk of self-neglect and suicide.
- Treat comorbid physical illnesses or substance misuse problems.

- For mild depression, self-help groups, structured physical activity groups, guided self-help or computerised cognitive behavioural therapy (CBT) are often helpful (Chapter 33).
- If these less intensive therapies do not help, individual CBT or interpersonal therapy (IPT) may be recommended. Behavioural activation or, where appropriate, behavioural couples therapy can also be of use.
- Psychological therapy should be given together with antidepressants (Chapter 35) for moderate or severe depression. These can have a 60–70% response rate but often fail because of inadequate dosage, duration or adherence.
- Continuing antidepressants for at least six months reduces relapse; in recurrent depression, prophylactic effects have been demonstrated for up to five years. When discontinuing antidepressants, taper slowly to avoid withdrawal symptoms. In bipolar depression, mood stabilisers (e.g. lithium – Chapter 36) are preferable. CBT or mindfulness-based cognitive therapy can also help prevent relapse.
- Resistant depression may respond to combining an antidepressant (augmenting) with lithium, an atypical antipsychotic (aripiprazole, olanzapine, risperidone, quetiapine) or another antidepressant (e.g. mirtazipine).
- Electroconvulsive therapy (ECT) is very effective in severe cases, particularly where psychosis or stupor is present, and can be lifesaving if fluids and food are being refused.

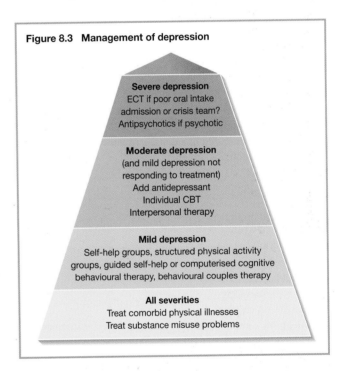

Figure 8.3 Management of depression

Severe depression
ECT if poor oral intake
admission or crisis team?
Antipsychotics if psychotic

Moderate depression
(and mild depression not responding to treatment)
Add antidepressant
Individual CBT
Interpersonal therapy

Mild depression
Self-help groups, structured physical activity groups, guided self-help or computerised cognitive behavioural therapy, behavioural couples therapy

All severities
Treat comorbid physical illnesses
Treat substance misuse problems

Prognosis

- Single episodes of depression usually last three to eight months. About 20% of patients remain depressed for two years or more and 50% have recurrences; this rises to 80% in severe cases. Recurrent episodes tend to become increasingly severe with shortening of disease-free periods, emphasising the importance of prophylactic treatment.
- Lifetime suicide risk is 15% in severe depression but much lower in milder illness. There is an association between major depressive disorder/bipolar disorder and increased cardiovascular morbidity and mortality. Predictors of poor outcome include early onset, greater symptom severity and psychiatric or physical comorbidity.

9 Bipolar Affective Disorder

Definitions and classification

Bipolar affective disorder (previously called manic depression) is characterised by recurrent episodes of altered mood and activity, involving both upswings and downswings. Classificatory systems (ICD-10, DSM-5) define individual episodes and patterns of recurrence.

Individual episodes are classified as:
- *depressive* (see Chapter 8)
- *manic*
- *hypomanic* (less severe and without psychotic symptoms)
- *mixed* (less usual) where features of both mania and major depression are present or alternate rapidly.
- In ICD-10, *bipolar affective disorder* is defined as at least two episodes, including at least one hypomanic or manic episode.
- In DSM-5, patterns of recurrence can be classified as:
  - *bipolar I disorder* – one or more manic or mixed episodes and usually one or more major depressive episodes;
  - *bipolar II disorder* – recurrent major depressive and hypomanic but not manic episodes;
  - *cyclothymic disorder* – chronic mood fluctuations over at least two years, with episodes of depression and hypomania (but not mania) of insufficient severity to meet diagnostic criteria.

Clinical features

The cardinal clinical feature of a manic or hypomanic episode is alteration in mood, which is usually elated and expansive but may also be characterised by intense irritability. DSM-5 emphasises changes in activity and energy as well as mood. Associated features include:
- increased psychomotor activity (distractibility, decreased need for sleep);
- exaggerated optimism;
- inflated self-esteem;
- decreased social inhibition, with apparent disregard for potentially harmful consequences of:
  - sexual overactivity
  - reckless spending
  - dangerous driving
  - inappropriate business, religious or political initiatives;
- heightened sensory awareness;
- rapid thinking and speech:
  - uninterruptible (pressured) speech
  - flight of ideas (Chapter 2).
- (in mania only) mood-congruent delusions and hallucinations, usually auditory.

Insight is often absent. Manic and hypomanic episodes are distinguished on the basis that hypomania is less severe, causing less disruption to work and social or interpersonal life, and psychotic symptoms are absent. Manic episodes have a median duration of four months. Depressive episodes tend to last longer (median six months). Recovery may or may not be complete between episodes.

Differential diagnosis

- Substance abuse (particularly amphetamines or cocaine).
- Mood abnormalities secondary to endocrine disturbance (idiopathic Cushing's syndrome or steroid-induced psychoses) or epilepsy.
- Schizophrenia: persecutory or grandiose delusions, auditory hallucinations and increased psychomotor activity may occur in both conditions.
- Schizoaffective disorder should be diagnosed where affective and schizophreniform symptoms (e.g. First Rank Symptoms – see Chapter 9) are equally prominent.
- Personality disorders (emotionally unstable or histrionic) may mimic some features of the mood or behavioural disturbance of mania and hypomania.
- Attention-deficit hyperactivity disorder (ADHD) in younger people and transient psychoses induced by extreme stress, although in both elevation of mood is rare.
- Bipolar disorder can also be comorbid with conditions including substance use, personality disorders, obsessive–compulsive disorder and anxiety.

Epidemiology

- Lifetime prevalences are:
  bipolar I disorder   1%
  bipolar II disorder   0.4–2%
  cyclothymia   2.5%.
- The female:male ratio is approximately equal for bipolar I disorder; some but not all studies show a female excess in the bipolar II group.
- Peak age of onset is in the early twenties. The illness often starts in childhood and adolescence. There may be a second smaller peak of onset in later life (45 to 54 years)
- Several studies have shown greater prevalence rates in higher social classes, probably reflecting differences in access to diagnosis.
- Black African and African Caribbean people are more likely to present with mania and to present with more severe psychotic symptoms than are white European people –social exclusion and late diagnosis, and thus treatment, have been suggested as reasons for this.

Aetiology

- There is evidence for a strong genetic component, with evidence of heritability of mood disorder from other family members in 60% or more people. The lifetime risk of bipolar disorder is increased in first degree relatives of a person with bipolar disorder (40–70% for a monozygotic twin; 5–10% for other first degree relatives). Autism, ADHD, bipolar disorder, major depression and schizophrenia share some of the same genetic risk factors.
- A number of studies have reported abnormalities in the hypothalamic-pituitary-adrenal (HPA) axis in bipolar disorder which are consistent with reduced HPA axis feedback – e.g. chronically elevated cortisol levels in depression

Psychiatry at a Glance, Sixth Edition. Cornelius Katona, Claudia Cooper, Mary Robertson. © 2016 John Wiley & Sons, Ltd. Published 2016 by John Wiley & Sons, Ltd.
Companion website: www.ataglanceseries.com/psychiatry

- The hypothalamic-pituitary-thyroid (HPT) axis is also implicated; approximately 25% of those with rapid cycling bipolar disorder have evidence of hypothyroidism
- Magnetic resonance imaging (MRI) findings include smaller prefrontal lobes and enlarged amygdala and globus pallidus. There may be diminished prefrontal modulation of subcortical and medial temporal structures (eg, amygdala, anterior striatum and thalamus) that results in dysregulation of mood.
- Prolonged psychosocial stressors during childhood, such as neglect or abuse, are associated with HPA axis dysfunction in later life, which may result in hypersensitivity to stress. People with a history of childhood sexual or physical abuse appear to be more at risk and to have a worse prognosis.
- There is a markedly increased risk of manic episodes in the early postpartum weeks; this may relate to dopamine receptor supersensitivity associated with postpartum falls in oestrogen and progesterone levels (Chapter 25).
- Sleep disturbance can induce mania. Disturbance of circadian rhythms (e.g. in jet lag and sleep loss) may precipitate an episode, as may a recent life event. There appears to be an increase in manic episodes in the spring and early summer.
- Psychodynamic models of mania suggest denial of loss or loss-associated conflict in order to avoid depression, or loss of super-ego ('conscience') control. These are not frequently invoked in mainstream psychiatry.

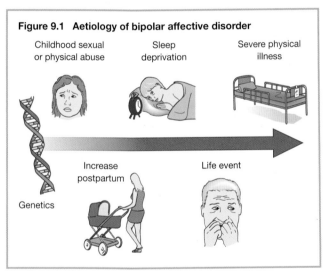

Figure 9.1 Aetiology of bipolar affective disorder

Childhood sexual or physical abuse

Sleep deprivation

Severe physical illness

Genetics

Increase postpartum

Life event

- 'Secondary' mania may be precipitated by severe physical illness, particularly stroke.

Management (NICE guideline 2014)

- A coordinated care programme, with rapid access to support at times of crisis, is essential. Hospitalisation is required for those at significant risk of harm.

Treating manic and hypomanic episodes

- Effective first line drugs for treatment of acute mania are haloperidol, olanzapine, quetiapine or risperidone.

- Lithium has a slower onset of action, but lithium or valproate can be considered if the first-line drugs above are ineffective. Benzodiazepines may be used in the short term for acute behavioural disturbance. Lorazepam and antipsychotics may be useful for rapid tranquillisation (see Chapter 34).

Treating depressive episodes

- Antidepressants may precipitate mania or 'rapid cycling' (with four or more episodes a year), so they should not be prescribed without an antimanic/mood-stabilising agent. If a patient is taking an antidepressant at the onset of an acute manic episode, the antidepressant should be stopped. For episodes of moderate or severe depression in bipolar disorder, 2014 NICE guidelines recommend quetiapine, olanzapine, lamotrigine or a combination of olanzapine and fluoxetine.

Treating bipolar affective disorder

- Structured psychological interventions (individual/family/group) should be offered.
- When planning long-term pharmacological treatment to prevent relapse, it is important to take into account drugs that have been effective during episodes of mania or bipolar depression.
- Discussions should include whether to continue this treatment or switch to lithium because lithium is the most effective long-term treatment for bipolar disorder. Lithium reduces the risk of suicide; it may also be useful in cyclothymia. Lithium therapy requires blood monitoring (see Chapter 36).
- Valproate, olanzapine and quetiapine are also effective treatments.
- Weight and cardiovascular and metabolic indicators of morbidity should be routinely monitored in people with bipolar disorder.
- The teratogenic toxicity associated with valproate severely limits its use in women of child-bearing potential. Lithium is also teratogenic.

Prognosis

- The lifetime prognosis following a single manic episode is poor, with 90% of patients having manic or depressive recurrences (averaging four episodes in 10 years). In bipolar I disorder, both the frequency and severity of episodes tend to increase for the first four or five episodes but then plateau.
- A minority who develop rapid cycling have a particularly poor prognosis and seldom respond to lithium. However, they respond better to antiepileptic mood stabilisers.
- Long-term functional prognosis (work, family, etc.) (particularly in untreated patients) is almost as poor as in schizophrenia.
- There is an overall increase in premature mortality, only partially explained by a suicide rate of 10%. Prognosis for bipolar II disorder is better, although there remains a high suicide risk.
- Cyclothymia runs a chronic course and approximately 30% of patients risk developing full-blown bipolar disorder.
- There is an association with violence that is almost completely explained by the greater risk of violence in those patients with comorbid substance misuse.

10 Stress Reactions (Including Bereavement)

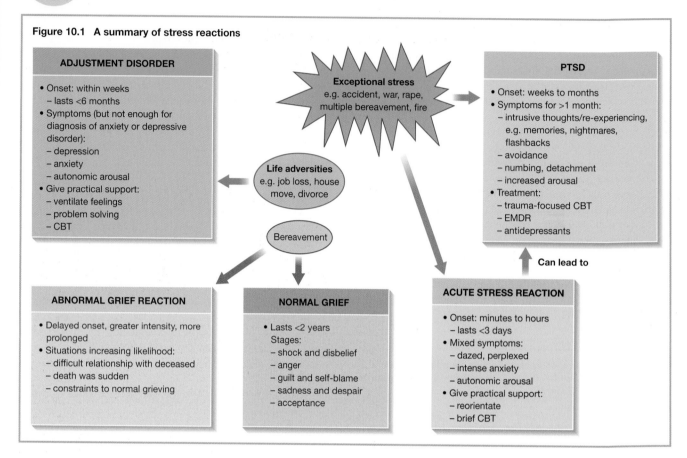

Figure 10.1 A summary of stress reactions

ADJUSTMENT DISORDER
- Onset: within weeks
  - lasts <6 months
- Symptoms (but not enough for diagnosis of anxiety or depressive disorder):
  - depression
  - anxiety
  - autonomic arousal
- Give practical support:
  - ventilate feelings
  - problem solving
  - CBT

Life adversities
e.g. job loss, house move, divorce

Exceptional stress
e.g. accident, war, rape, multiple bereavement, fire

Bereavement

PTSD
- Onset: weeks to months
- Symptoms for >1 month:
  - intrusive thoughts/re-experiencing, e.g. memories, nightmares, flashbacks
  - avoidance
  - numbing, detachment
  - increased arousal
- Treatment:
  - trauma-focused CBT
  - EMDR
  - antidepressants

Can lead to

ABNORMAL GRIEF REACTION
- Delayed onset, greater intensity, more prolonged
- Situations increasing likelihood:
  - difficult relationship with deceased
  - death was sudden
  - constraints to normal grieving

NORMAL GRIEF
- Lasts <2 years
  Stages:
  - shock and disbelief
  - anger
  - guilt and self-blame
  - sadness and despair
  - acceptance

ACUTE STRESS REACTION
- Onset: minutes to hours
  - lasts <3 days
- Mixed symptoms:
  - dazed, perplexed
  - intense anxiety
  - autonomic arousal
- Give practical support:
  - reorientate
  - brief CBT

Major psychological stress involves threat or loss. Reactions to a broad range of major stressors (physical or sexual assault, transport accidents, natural disasters, war) are often similar in nature and involve:
- emotional responses (fear from threat and sadness at loss);
- physical symptoms (autonomic arousal and/or fatigue);
- psychological responses, which may be conscious (e.g. avoidance behaviour) or unconscious (e.g. denial or dissociation).

Abnormal stress reactions represent exaggerated or maladaptive responses. They may be acute and self-limiting (acute stress reactions) or prolonged (post-traumatic stress disorder [PTSD], adjustment disorder or abnormal grief).

Acute stress reactions
- ICD-10 criteria for acute stress reactions require rapid onset (within minutes or hours) of extreme responses to sudden and severe stressful events.
- There is a mixed and usually changing picture of symptoms that include:
  - an initial state of feeling dazed or perplexed;
  - depression, anger, despair;
  - purposeless overactivity and withdrawal;
  - intense subjective anxiety with autonomic arousal (sweating, dry mouth, tachycardia, vomiting);

- dissociative symptoms, which predict increased risk of PTSD, include wandering aimlessly;
  - reduced sleep and nightmares.
- Initial management involves:
  - helping to reorient and 'ground' the individual;
  - practical support (e.g. temporary housing following a natural disaster);
  - brief cognitive behavioural therapy (CBT) to improve outcome and reduce the rate of chronic PTSD.
- There is no evidence that anxiolytics or hypnotics are effective, and they carry a risk of dependence.
- In most cases symptoms resolve rapidly (within a few hours at the most) where removal from the stressful environment is possible. If the stress continues or cannot by its nature be reversed, the symptoms usually begin to diminish after 24 to 48 hours and are minimal after about three days.
- Persistence of symptoms for more than one month indicates the development of PTSD.

Adjustment disorders
- Adjustment disorders include a range of abnormal psychological responses to life adversity (e.g. job loss, house move or divorce).

- The onset is usually within weeks of the stressful event and the duration less than six months, unless there are factors leading to persistence (e.g. ongoing litigation). Adjustment disorders usually improve following resolution of their precipitating cause.
- The presentation includes a broad mix of symptoms of anxiety (autonomic arousal, insomnia, irritability) and depression (sadness, tearfulness, worry). The diagnosis should be made only where there are insufficient symptoms to justify a diagnosis of a specific anxiety or depressive disorder.
- Initial management may involve encouragement to ventilate feelings and to develop appropriate problem-solving strategies. Sometimes formal CBT is required.
- Adjustment to chronic or terminal illness may manifest as anxiety, depression or exaggerated disability. There may be a sequence (similar to that in bereavement) of:

shock and denial (search for cure) ⇒ anger ⇒ sadness ⇒ acceptance

Management involves adequate symptomatic control (particularly of pain), honest explanation, supportive psychotherapy and family counselling.

PTSD

- The onset of PTSD follows a severe stressful experience that is of an exceptionally threatening or catastrophic nature; this can include assault, accident, disaster, act of terrorism or battle. It may occur in adults or children. ICD-10 states that onset is usually within six months of stressor (although it may rarely exceed this); DSM-5 that symptoms persist for at least one month.
- The characteristic features of PTSD involve:
  - *persistent intrusive thinking or re-experiencing* of the trauma, such as traumatic memories, recurrent dreams or nightmares and re-enactments ('flashbacks') of the traumatic event;
  - *avoidance* of reminders of the event (e.g. the scene of an accident), and thoughts, feelings and conversations associated with the trauma;
  - *numbing, detachment and estrangement* from others, *loss of interest* in significant activities and sense of a foreshortened future;
  - *increased arousal* with autonomic symptoms, hypervigilance, sleep disturbance, irritability, poor concentration and exaggerated startle response.
- Alcohol or substance misuse may be a symptom and/or long-term complication.
- Depression may be comorbid or secondary to PTSD.
- Risk for PTSD is proportional to the magnitude of the stressor but may be greater following man-made rather than natural disasters and if some stress continues. Lack of social support, the presence of other adversities at the time of the trauma and premorbid personality are vulnerability factors.
- Effective treatments include:
  - trauma-focused CBT;
  - eye movement desensitisation and reprocessing therapy (EMDR; see Chapter 33);
  - antidepressant drugs (e.g. paroxetine or miratzapine) – these have been shown to be effective but should not be used first line unless patients do not wish to engage in psychological treatment.
- Debriefing is no longer indicated because it does not, as previously thought, prevent PTSD (in debriefing, patients were encouraged to recall the stressful events in detail soon after the trauma and were then supported through the associated emotions.)

- Many PTSD victims recover over the first few months. If the syndrome persists over one to two years, it may become chronic, possibly for the rest of a victim's life, as with many Holocaust survivors.

Bereavement and grief

- Bereavement is associated with increased mortality (from cardiovascular disease and cancer) and may precipitate depression and even suicide.
- **'Normal'** grief may last up to two years. The classic stages of grieving are:

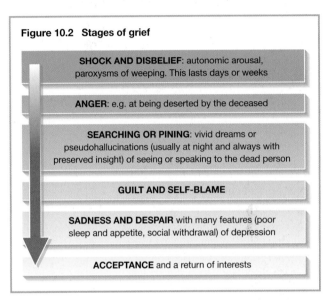

Figure 10.2 Stages of grief

SHOCK AND DISBELIEF: autonomic arousal, paroxysms of weeping. This lasts days or weeks

ANGER: e.g. at being deserted by the deceased

SEARCHING OR PINING: vivid dreams or pseudohallucinations (usually at night and always with preserved insight) of seeing or speaking to the dead person

GUILT AND SELF-BLAME

SADNESS AND DESPAIR with many features (poor sleep and appetite, social withdrawal) of depression

ACCEPTANCE and a return of interests

- The sequence of stages is often less clear-cut than this linear model suggests. Bereavement may be characterised by jumbled feelings as people pass in and out of these stages.
- Normal grieving requires no specific management apart from support and encouragement to ventilate feelings and accept them as normal. Symptoms often recur briefly on anniversaries.
- **'Abnormal'** grief is characterised by delayed onset, greater intensity of symptoms or prolongation of the reaction. Suicidal ideas may be harboured during abnormal pining (a wish to be with the deceased) or despair.
- In ICD-10, abnormal grief reaction is coded as an adjustment disorder. DSM-5 lists persistent complex bereavement disorder as a disorder for further study, and a separate diagnostic category is also being considered for ICD-11. It is more likely where:
  - the relationship with the deceased was problematic (ambivalent or overinvolved);
  - the death was sudden;
  - normal grieving was impeded by social constraints (e.g. 'putting on a brave face for the children').
- Abnormal grief reactions last longer than normal grief – at least six months after the bereavement. Symptoms are intense and disabling, including:
  - confusion about one's role in life or diminished sense of self, feeling life is empty since the loss or that it is difficult to move on;
  - feeling numb, stunned or shocked since the loss, or feeling angry or struggling to accepting it.
- Abnormal grief may respond to CBT, encouraging structured review of the relationship and giving vent to the emotions produced. Complex bereavement or adjustment disorder should not be diagnosed if criteria for depressive disorder are met.

11 Anxiety Disorders

Anxiety

- Anxiety is an unpleasant emotional state involving subjective fear, bodily discomfort and physical symptoms. There is often a feeling of impending threat or death, which may or may not be in response to a recognisable threat.
- The Yerkes–Dodson curve shows that anxiety can be beneficial up to a plateau of optimal function, beyond which, with increasing anxiety, performance deteriorates.

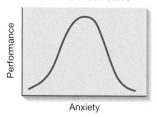

Yerkes–Dodson curve

Anxiety disorders

- Pathological anxiety can involve:
  - generalised anxiety, as in generalised anxiety disorder (GAD);
  - discrete anxiety attacks caused by an external stimulus (in phobias) or without external stimulus (in panic disorder).
- Anxiety disorders may present alone but are also frequently comorbid with other disorders including depression, substance misuse or another anxiety disorder.
- Anxiety occurs in other disorders such as depression.

Epidemiology

- Around 6% of the general population have an anxiety disorder at one time. The anxiety disorders comprise:
  - generalised anxiety disorder (GAD) (2–4%)
  - panic disorder (1%)
  - phobias (agoraphobia, social phobia, specific phobias)
  - obsessive–compulsive disorder (Chapter 12).
- Anxiety disorders are more common in women, younger adults and the middle-aged.
- Lower rates are reported in young men and older people. In older people this may be because of the difficulty in detecting anxiety in old age using standard measures.

Aetiology
Biological

- Low levels of GABA, a neurotransmitter that reduces activity in the central nervous system, contribute to anxiety.
- Mouse studies have found that the frontal cortex and amygdala undergo structural remodelling induced by the stress of maternal separation and isolation, which alters behavioural and physiological responses in adulthood.
- Heightened amygdala activation occurs in response to disorder-relevant stimuli in post-traumatic stress disorder, social phobia and specific phobia.

- The medial prefrontal cortex, insula and hippocampus have also been implicated.
- Alcohol and benzodiazepine abuse can worsen or cause anxiety and panic attacks.

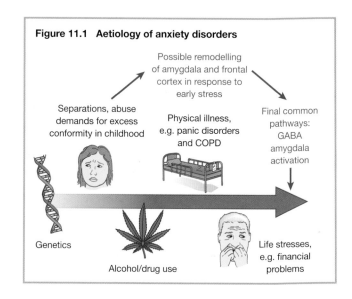

Figure 11.1 Aetiology of anxiety disorders

Genetics

- First degree relatives of people with an anxiety disorder have a quadrupled risk of developing an anxiety disorder.
- Some of this risk is disorder-specific and some is not.
  - The genetic factors of panic attacks appear to overlap with depression by about 50%.
  - GAD and depression are genetically related.
- For social phobia and agoraphobia, genetic risk appears to be mainly due to inheritance of personality traits (low extraversion and high neuroticism).
- Inheritance of specific phobias appears to be independent of personality.

Childhood

- There is an association with childhood abuse, separations, demands for high achievement and excessive conformity.

Stress

- Anxiety disorder can arise in response to life stresses such as financial problems or chronic disease.
- Anxiety disorders are precipitated and perpetuated by physical health problems:
  - a degree of anxiety when facing physical illness, especially when the diagnosis is unclear, is normal;
  - concerns about incontinence or being ill when out may perpetuate agoraphobia;
  - Panic disorder is 10 times more common in people with chronic obstructive airways disease, probably because breathlessness precipitates the symptoms of panic (see Figure 11.2).

Panic disorder

- Recurrent episodic severe panic (anxiety) attacks, which occur unpredictably and are not restricted to any particular situation.
- Panic attacks are discrete periods of intense fear, impending doom or discomfort accompanied by characteristic symptoms:
    - palpitations, tachycardia
    - sweating, trembling, breathlessness
    - feeling of choking
    - chest pain/discomfort
    - nausea/abdominal discomfort
    - dizziness, paraesthesia
    - chills and hot flushes
    - derealisation/depersonalisation (Chapter 2)
    - fear of losing control, 'going crazy' or dying.
- Typically, they only last a few minutes.
- 'Anticipatory fear' of having a panic attack may develop, with consequent reluctance to be alone away from home. DSM-5 states that for panic disorder to be diagnosed, panic attacks must be followed by at least a month of persistent worry about having another attack or maladaptive behavioural changes related to the attack.
- According to the cognitive model, panic attacks occur when catastrophic misinterpretations of ambiguous physical sensations (such as shortness of breath or increased heart rate) increase arousal, creating a positive feedback loop that results in panic.

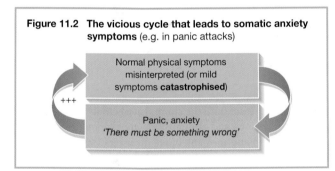

Figure 11.2 The vicious cycle that leads to somatic anxiety symptoms (e.g. in panic attacks)

- Selective serotonin reuptake inhibitors (SSRIs) (Chapter 35) and cognitive behavioural therapy (CBT) (Chapter 33) or self-help materials based on CBT principles are recommended first-line treatments.
- Tricyclic antidepressants (imipramine and clomipramine) may be helpful where SSRIs are ineffective.
- Benzodiazepines are not recommended.

Generalised anxiety disorder (GAD)

- GAD is characterised by generalised, persistent, excessive anxiety or worry (apprehensive expectation) about a number of events (e.g. work, school performance) that the individual finds difficult to control, lasting for at least three weeks (according to ICD-10) or six months or longer (according to DSM-5). The anxiety is usually associated with:
    - subjective apprehension (fears, worries),
    - increased vigilance,
    - feeling restless and on edge,
    - sleeping difficulties (initial/middle insomnia, fatigue on waking),
    - motor tension (tremor, hyperactive deep reflexes),
    - autonomic hyperactivity (e.g. tachycardia).
- GAD may be comorbid with other anxiety disorders, depression, alcohol and drug abuse.

- Differential diagnoses include:
    - withdrawal from drugs or alcohol,
    - excessive caffeine consumption,
    - depression,
    - psychotic disorders,
    - organic causes such as thyrotoxicosis, parathyroid disease, hypoglycaemia, phaeochromocytoma and carcinoid syndrome.
- Treatment with individual guided self-help (CBT principles) and psychoeducational groups often helps.
- If not or if symptoms are more severe, the next step is face-to-face CBT or applied relaxation.
- SSRIs or serotonin noradrenaline reuptake inhibitors (SNRIs) are the recommended pharmacological treatments where these are required. Pregabalin is sometimes used as a second-line treatment.
- CBT (self-help material or face-to-face) for GAD seeks to:
    - identify morbid anticipatory thoughts and replace them with more realistic cognitions
    - learn and use distraction, breathing and relaxation exercises.

Benzodiazepines should only be used in crises and usually not beyond two to four weeks.

Phobic disorders
Agoraphobia

- Agoraphobia is often comorbid with panic disorder and is characterised by fear and avoidance of places or situations from which escape may be difficult or in which help may not be available in the event of having a panic attack.
- Diagnosis requires that anxiety is restricted to being in the following situations that are therefore avoided:
    - crowds
    - public places
    - travelling away from home
    - travelling alone.
- Some people with marked agoraphobia experience paradoxically little anxiety because they avoid all phobic situations. They may, for example, leave the house only occasionally to visit a very restricted number of places.
- CBT is considered the mainstay of treatment and usually involves graded exposure to avoided situations (see Chapter 33), but SSRIs are also effective. Treatment response depends on the patient's engagement with treatment and motivation for change.

Social phobia

- Social phobia is prevalent and treatable.
- It is equally common in men and women. Onset is usually by mid-adolescence, but affected individuals often do not seek help for many years.
- It is characterised by a persistent fear of social situations in which the individual is exposed to unfamiliar people or to possible scrutiny by others and fears that he or she will be humiliated or embarrassed (e.g. by blushing, shaking, vomiting).
- Management includes CBT, self-help materials, graded self-exposure and social skills training. Drug treatments should not be first line but, if psychosocial treatment fails or the patient does not want it, may help. SSRIs are most commonly used.

Specific phobias

- Specific phobias are characterised by fear of specific people, objects or situations (e.g. flying, heights, animals, blood).
- Treatment is typically by graded exposure therapy and response prevention. Short-term use of benzodiazepines may be helpful if the phobia is only rarely encountered (e.g. flying twice a year).

(12) Obsessions and Compulsions

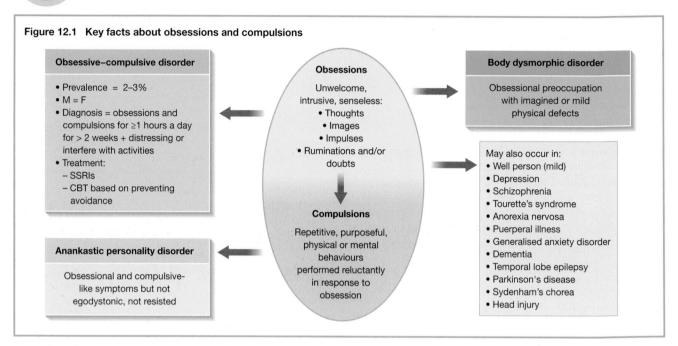

Figure 12.1 Key facts about obsessions and compulsions

Obsessive–compulsive disorder

• Prevalence = 2–3%
• M = F
• Diagnosis = obsessions and compulsions for ≥1 hours a day for > 2 weeks + distressing or interfere with activities
• Treatment:
– SSRIs
– CBT based on preventing avoidance

Anankastic personality disorder

Obsessional and compulsive-like symptoms but not egodystonic, not resisted

Obsessions

Unwelcome, intrusive, senseless:
• Thoughts
• Images
• Impulses
• Ruminations and/or doubts

Compulsions

Repetitive, purposeful, physical or mental behaviours performed reluctantly in response to obsession

Body dysmorphic disorder

Obsessional preoccupation with imagined or mild physical defects

May also occur in:
• Well person (mild)
• Depression
• Schizophrenia
• Tourette's syndrome
• Anorexia nervosa
• Puerperal illness
• Generalised anxiety disorder
• Dementia
• Temporal lobe epilepsy
• Parkinson's disease
• Sydenham's chorea
• Head injury

Obsessions and compulsions

Obsessions are unwelcome, persistent, recurrent, intrusive, senseless and uncomfortable for the individual, who attempts to suppress or neutralise them and recognises them as absurd (egodystonic) and a product of his or her own mind. Obsessions may be:
• thoughts (e.g. blasphemy, sex, violence, contamination, numbers);
• images (vivid, morbid or violent scenes);
• impulses (e.g. a fear of jumping in front of a train);
• ruminations (continuous pondering);
• doubts.
Obsessions should be distinguished from volitional fantasies (thoughts that are not displeasurable (egosyntonic)).
Compulsions are repetitive, purposeful physical or mental behaviours performed with reluctance in response to an obsession. They are carried out according to certain rules in a stereotyped fashion and are designed to neutralise or prevent discomfort or a dreaded event. The activity is excessive and not connected to the triggering thought (obsession) in a realistic way. The individual realises the behaviour is unreasonable. Compulsions include:
• hand-washing, cleaning;
• counting, checking;
• touching and rearrangement of objects to achieve symmetry;
• mental compulsions (e.g. checking and repeating thoughts);
• hoarding;
• arithmomania (counting);
• onomatomania (the desire to utter a forbidden word);
• folie du pourquoi
• (the irresistible habit of seeking explanations for commonplace facts by asking endless questions);
• inappropriate and excessive tidiness.

Compulsions should be distinguished from rituals and 'normal' superstitious behaviour (actions that have a magical quality and are culturally sanctioned, such as touching wood for good luck). If resistance to the obsessions or compulsions is attempted, anxiety usually increases until the compulsive activity is performed.

Mild obsessions and compulsions are common in the general population and in many other disorders (see Figure 12.1). Recent evidence suggests that there is comorbidity between the spectrum of obsessive–compulsive disorders and a range of other psychiatric disorders including bipolar affective disorder, Tourette's syndrome, pathological gambling and hypochondriasis.

Obsessive–compulsive disorder (OCD)
Clinical characteristics

• OCD is characterised by time-consuming (>1 hour/day) obsessions and/or compulsions. An ICD-10 diagnosis of OCD requires that obsessions or compulsions are present most days for at least two weeks, are distressing and interfere with activities.
• Avoidance of stimuli or activities that trigger obsessive–compulsive symptoms is very common. Resistance is characteristic but may not persist.
• Onset is usually during adolescence.
• OCD can be divided into four subtypes, characterised by:
  • obsessions and compulsions (usually hand-washing) concerned with contamination (most common subtype);
  • checking compulsions in response to obsessional thoughts about potential harm (e.g. leaving the gas on);
  • obsessions without overt compulsive acts;
  • hoarding (the acquisition of, and difficulty in discarding, items that appear worthless to others).

Psychiatry at a Glance, Sixth Edition. Cornelius Katona, Claudia Cooper, Mary Robertson. © 2016 John Wiley & Sons, Ltd. Published 2016 by John Wiley & Sons, Ltd.
Companion website: www.ataglanceseries.com/psychiatry

• Complications include depression and abuse of anxiolytics or alcohol. Severe OCD can lead to as much distress and functional impairment as psychotic illness.

Epidemiology

The lifetime prevalence of OCD in the general population is 2–3%. Men and women are affected equally.

Aetiology

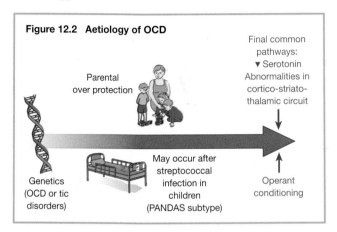

Figure 12.2 Aetiology of OCD

Final common pathways:
▼ Serotonin
Abnormalities in cortico-striato-thalamic circuit

Parental over protection

Genetics (OCD or tic disorders)

May occur after streptococcal infection in children (PANDAS subtype)

Operant conditioning

• People with OCD are more likely to have a family history of OCD (50% of cases), tics or Tourette's syndrome.
• Some studies report an association with parental overprotection.
• Biochemical abnormalities (especially involving serotonin) are now thought to be important in the pathophysiology of OCD.
• OCD may be caused by an abnormality of the cortico-striatothalamic circuit, which mediates social behaviour. A fundamental problem appears to be an inability to inhibit or suppress inappropriate mental or physical acts. Neuroimaging has shown functional abnormalities in the frontal cortex and basal ganglia.
• Psychoanalytic theories view OCD as a defence against cruel and aggressive fantasies (filling the mind with obsessional thoughts prevents undesirable ideas entering consciousness) and defensive regression to the anal stage of development.
• Behavioural theories propose that compulsive behaviour is learned and maintained by operant conditioning processes, the anxiety reduction following the compulsive behaviour strengthening, and ultimately increasing, the need to perform the compulsion in response to an obsessional thought.
• OCD and related tic disorders may occur suddenly in children. These were known as paediatric autoimmune neuropsychiatric disorders associated with streptococci (PANDAS), but doubt has been cast more recently on the relationship between streptococcus and the behaviours. More recently the terms 'childhood/paediatric acute neuropsychiatric syndrome' (CANS/PANS) have evolved to describe these acute onset disorders without defining aetiology.

Body dysmorphic disorder (BDD)

• This disorder (also called dysmorphophobia) is characterised by a preoccupation with an imagined defect in appearance or markedly excessive concern with a slight physical anomaly.
• Time-consuming behaviours include mirror-gazing, comparing particular features with those of others, excessive camouflaging tactics to hide the defect, skin-picking and reassurance-seeking; the sufferer may even request surgery.
• Around 0.5% of the general population have BDD.
• It is related to OCD and hypochondriacal disorder.

Management of OCD and BDD

• Psychoeducation helps people understand their disorder.
• First-line treatment is with cognitive behavioural therapy (CBT), together with medication.
• CBT involves *exposure* followed by *response prevention*; the patient is encouraged not to perform the unwanted compulsive behaviour (e.g. hand-washing) while simultaneously being exposed to a situation associated with it (e.g. wiping a toilet seat). CBT can be self-help, group or individual therapy.

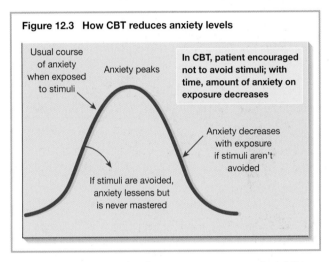

Figure 12.3 How CBT reduces anxiety levels

Usual course of anxiety when exposed to stimuli

Anxiety peaks

In CBT, patient encouraged not to avoid stimuli; with time, amount of anxiety on exposure decreases

Anxiety decreases with exposure if stimuli aren't avoided

If stimuli are avoided, anxiety lessens but is never mastered

• Drug treatment is with selective serotonin reuptake inhibitors (SSRIs) or clomipramine. These drugs are effective even in the absence of coexistent depressive symptomatology. They may take up to 12 weeks to have an effect.
• Neuroimaging studies show that similar changes in the caudate nucleus occur in response to both CBT and to SSRIs. Overall response to CBT and/or drugs is about 75%; in contrast, placebo responses in clinical trials are low (5%).
• Psychosurgery (cingulotomy, capsulotomy) is very rarely used but may be effective in the most severe and treatment-resistant cases. Deep brain stimulation (see Chapter 37) has been used successfully recently, but in a small, select number of patients.

Course and prognosis

• OCD may follow an episodic or chronic course. Patients with prominent compulsions, comorbid tic disorders, persistent life stresses or premorbid anankastic personality fare worst.
• Traditionally, OCD was thought to carry a low risk of suicide; recent research, however, contradicts this.

Anankastic personality disorder

• Also called 'obsessive–compulsive personality disorder'.
• Characteristic features include:
  • rigidity of thinking,
  • perfectionism that may interfere with completing tasks,
  • moralistic preoccupation with rules,
  • excessive cleanliness and orderliness,
  • objectively high standards that are seldom achieved,
  • a tendency to hoard,
  • emotional coldness.
• These are egosyntonic life traits with no obvious onset.

13 Eating Disorders

Figure 13.1 Comparison of anorexia nervosa and bulimia nervosa

	Anorexia nervosa	Bulimia nervosa
Definition	• Morbid fear of fatness • Distorted body image, • Deliberate weight loss • Amenorrhoea • BMI < 17.5	• Morbid fear of fatness, distorted body image • Craving for food and uncontrolled binge-eating • Purging/vomiting/laxative abuse • Fluctuating (normal or excessive) weight
Epidemiology	Onset at age 13–20 – men later Prevalence 1–2% in schoolgirls and female students Sex ratio F:M = 3:1	Onset usually at age 15–30 Prevalence 1–3% Sex ratio F:M = 3:1
Differential diagnosis	Psychosis: schizophrenia (delusions about food) Organic: diabetes (which may coexist with anorexia nervosa), Addison's, malabsorption, malignancy (all unlikely)	Psychiatric: Anorexia nervosa Neurological: Kleine–Levin, Klüver–Bucy

Management	• Family interventions
	• Motivational counselling
	• CBT/IPT
	• Hospitalisation if
	  – signficant physical abnormalities
	  – suicide risk
	  – BMI < 13.5
		• CBT/IPT
		• SSRIs (less effective than CBT)

Prognosis	• 40% recover • 35% improve • 20% develop chronic disorder • 5% death • Long-term risk of osteoporosis	Poor if • Low BMI • High frequency of purging • 30–40% remission with CBT/IPT

People with **anorexia nervosa** restrict what they eat and may compulsively overexercise to maintain an excessively low body weight. People with **bulimia nervosa** have intense cravings, secretively overeat, and then try to prevent weight gain (e.g. by vomiting). There is an important overlap. Some people with mixed symptoms are diagnosed with **eating disorder not otherwise specified**.

Epidemiology

• Anorexia and bulimia nervosa are three times more common in women. In childhood anorexia the sex ratio is nearly equal.
• Eating disorders usually begin in adolescence or early adulthood. Bulimia has a later onset (typically 18–19 years).
• Prevalence rates in young women are:
  • 1–2% for anorexia nervosa
  • 1–3% for bulimia nervosa.

Aetiological factors
Genetics

• Twin studies indicate a genetic component. First degree relatives have increased rates of eating disorders, anxiety disorders including OCD, depression, obsessional personality and (in bulimia) alcohol and substance abuse.

Personality

• Anxious, obsessive–compulsive and depressive traits and low self-esteem are common.

• People with anorexia often have constricted affect and reduced emotional expressiveness. Those with bulimia tend to be impulsive.

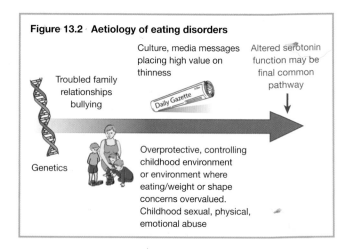

Figure 13.2 Aetiology of eating disorders

Troubled family relationships bullying

Culture, media messages placing high value on thinness

Altered serotonin function may be final common pathway

Genetics

Overprotective, controlling childhood environment or environment where eating/weight or shape concerns overvalued. Childhood sexual, physical, emotional abuse

Biological

• Altered brain serotonin (5-HT) function contributes to dysregulation of appetite, mood and impulse control.

Childhood environment

• Sexual, physical or emotional abuse.
• An overprotective or overcontrolling environment, or one where food, eating, weight or body shape are overvalued.

Psychiatry at a Glance, Sixth Edition. Cornelius Katona, Claudia Cooper, Mary Robertson. © 2016 John Wiley & Sons, Ltd. Published 2016 by John Wiley & Sons, Ltd.
Companion website: www.ataglanceseries.com/psychiatry

- Troubled interpersonal or family relationships.
- Being ridiculed because of size or weight.

Culture

Cultures that place a high value on being thin and consequent media messages/adverts encouraging dieting may contribute.

Anorexia nervosa

- There are 'restrictive' (minimal food intake and exercise) and 'bulimic' (episodic binge-eating with laxative use and induced vomiting) subtypes.
  - **Diagnosis** (ICD-10/DSM-5) requires:
    - a morbid fear of fatness;
    - deliberate weight loss;
    - distorted body image;
    - Body Mass Index (BMI, weight [kg]/ht [m]2) <17.5;
    - amenorrhoea (primary prepubertally, or secondary; oral contraceptive pill may still cause vaginal bleeds);
    - loss of sexual interest and potency in men; in prepubertal boys development will be arrested.
  - **Associated clinical features** include:
    - preoccupation with food (dieting, preparation of elaborate meals for others);
    - self-consciousness about eating in public, socially isolating behavior;
    - vigorous exercise;
    - constipation;
    - cold intolerance;
    - depressive and obsessive–compulsive symptoms.
  - **Physical signs/complications** include:
    - emaciation: often disguised by make-up/clothes;
    - dry and yellow skin;
    - fine lanugo hair on the face and trunk;
    - bradycardia and hypotension;
    - anaemia and leucopenia;
    - consequences of repeated vomiting, including hypokalaemia, alkalosis, pitted teeth, parotid swelling and scarring of the dorsum of the hand (Russell's sign).
  - **Differential diagnosis**
    - Organic causes of low weight (e.g. diabetes mellitus), which are not usually associated with abnormal attitudes to weight or eating. Diabetes may, however, coexist with anorexia.
    - Psychiatric causes of low weight include depression (which may also coexist with anorexia), psychotic disorders with delusions concerning food, and substance or alcohol abuse.
  - **Management**
    - Patients value their emaciated state and are usually ambivalent about treatment. Good therapeutic rapport and motivational counselling are important.
    - Exclude other diagnoses and monitor physical health.
    - For adolescents, family interventions are first line.
    - For adults, effective psychological therapies include cognitive behavioural therapy (CBT), interpersonal psychotherapy (IPT), focal psychodynamic therapy and family therapy (Chapter 33).
    - Specialist inpatient programmes typically provide a structured, symptom-focused treatment regime to achieve weight restoration. In very severe cases, nasogastric feeding may be instigated without the patient's consent under the Mental Health Act.
    - Coexistent depression should improve with weight gain, even without antidepressants.

- Treatment is usually as an outpatient but hospitalisation may be needed because of:
  - severe or rapid weight loss, or BMI <13.5, because of high risk of fatal arrhythmia or hypoglycaemia
  - significant suicide risk
  - physical sequelae of starvation or purging.
- **Prognosis**
  - Anorexia has the highest death rate of any psychiatric disorder (see Figure 13.1 for prognosis).
  - Osteoporosis is a long-term complication.

Bulimia nervosa

- **Diagnosis** (ICD-10/DSM-5) requires the presence of:
  - a morbid fear of fatness;
  - craving for food and binge-eating (of large amounts in a short time (e.g. >2000 kcal in a session));
  - recurrent behaviours to prevent weight gain (e.g. self-induced vomiting; misuse of laxatives, diuretics, enemas; omitting insulin; if diabetic; fasting or excessive exercise);
  - preoccupation with body weight and shape.
  - episodes are not exclusively during episodes of anorexia nervosa.
- **Associated clinical features** include:
  - normal or excessive weight (which often fluctuates);
  - loss of control or in a trance-like state during bingeing;
  - intense self-loathing and associated depression;
  - in 'multi-impulsive bulimia', alcohol and drug misuse, deliberate self-harm, stealing and/or sexual disinhibition coexist; poor impulse control is the common pathology.
- **Physical signs/complications** include:
  - amenorrhoea, which occurs in 50% (despite normal weight);
  - hypokalaemia, which may cause dysrhythmias or renal damage;
  - signs of excessive vomiting; acute oesophageal tears can occur during forced vomiting.
- **Differential diagnosis**
  - Consider anorexia nervosa, affective disorder and obesity.
  - Rare causes of overeating include Kleine–Levin and Klüver–Bucy syndromes (see Glossary).
- **Management** involves:
  - medical stabilisation;
  - psychotherapy (usually CBT or IPT) to establish a regular eating programme, re-establish control of diet and address underlying abnormal cognitions;
  - antidepressants; these are effective, best established for fluoxetine (60 mg) but less effective than CBT.
- **Prognosis**
  - With CBT or IPT, 30–40% achieve remission, gains which are typically maintained.

Binge-eating disorder and obesity

- This involves binge-eating with associated subjective loss of control and distress, without purging, and typically leads to obesity (BMI >30).
- Aetiological factors of **obesity** include:
  - weight-controlling genes
  - family and cultural influences
  - high availability of cheap calorific foods
  - a sedentary lifestyle.
- Management involves CBT, exercise and educational programmes. Anti-obesity medications such as orlistat (reduces absorption of dietary fat) are of short-term benefit. Surgery (e.g. gastric banding or bypass surgery) is indicated in severe cases.

14 Personality Disorders

Figure 14.1 The clusters of personality disorders

Cluster A (odd/eccentric)	Cluster B (flamboyant/dramatic)	Cluster C (fearful/anxious)
PARANOID PD • Cold affect • Pervasive distrust and suspiciousness • Preoccupied by mistrust of friends or spouse • Reluctance to confide • Bearing grudges • Interprets remarks negatively • Hypersensitivity to rebuffs • Grandiose sense of personal rights	**BORDERLINE (DSM)/EMOTIONALLY UNSTABLE (ICD)** • Unstable and intense interpersonal relationships, self-image, affect • Self-damaging impulsivity (spending, sex, substance abuse, reckless driving, binge-eating) • Identity confusion • Chronic anhedonia • Recurrent suicidal or self-mutilating behaviour • Transient paranoid ideation • Frantic efforts to avoid real/imagined abandonment	**DSM: AVOIDANT PD** **ICD: ANXIOUS PD** • Persistent feelings of tension and inadequacy • Social inhibitions • Unwillingness to become involved with people unless certain of being liked • Restriction in lifestyle to maintain physical security
SCHIZOID PD • Social withdrawal • Restricted range of emotional expression • Restricted pleasure, including in sex • Lacking confidants • Indifference to praise or criticism • Aloofness • Insensitivity to social norms	**HISTRIONIC PD** • Excessive shallow emotionality • Attention-seeking • Suggestibility • Shallow/labile affect • Inappropriate sexual seductiveness but immaturity • Narcissism • Grandiosity • Exploitative actions **DSM ONLY: NARCISSISTIC PD** • Pervasive grandiosity • Lack of empathy • Excessive need for praise	**DEPENDENT PD** • Excessive need to be taken care of, leading to submissive and clinging behaviour • Fear of separation • Needing excessive advice to make daily decisions • Needing others to assume responsibility • Difficulty in expressing disagreement for fear of loss of support/approval • Difficulty initiating projects because of low self-confidence • Goes to lengths to gain support from others • Constantly needs close relationships • Undue compliance with other's wishes • Unwilling to make demands on people • Preoccupation with fears of being left alone
SCHIZOTYPAL PD • Pervasive social and interpersonal deficits • Ideas of reference • Magical thinking • Unusual perception (e.g. bodily illusions) • Vague, circumstantial, tangential thinking • Inappropriate/constricted affect • Eccentricity, suspiciousness • Excessive social anxiety	**ANTISOCIAL (DSM)/DISSOCIAL (ICD)** • Persistent disregard for the rights or safety of others • Gross irresponsibility • Incapacity for maintaining relationships • Irritability • Low threshold for frustration and aggression • Incapacity for experiencing guilt or profiting from experience • Deceitfulness • Impulsivity • Disregard for personal safety • Proneness to blame others	**ANANKASTIC (DSM)/OBSESSIVE–COMPULSIVE (ICD) PD** • Excessive doubt, caution, rigidity and stubbornness • Preoccupation with details, rules, lists, order • Perfectionism interfering with task completion • Excessive conscientiousness • Preoccupation with productivity to the exclusion of pleasure and interpersonal relationships • Excessive pedantry and adherence to social norms • Unreasonable insistence that others submit to their way of doing things • Obsessional thoughts or impulses (without resistance)

Definition

• Personality disorders (PDs) are deeply ingrained and enduring patterns of behaviour that are abnormal in a particular culture, lead to subjective distress and sometimes cause others distress.
• PDs normally start in childhood or adolescence.
• The original distinction between PDs (lifelong and not treatable) and mental illnesses (briefer and treatable) is now less clear. People can recover from PDs, and there are now effective treatments for borderline PD.

Epidemiology

• In the adult population, PD of at least mild severity occurs in:
  • 5% of the general population
  • 20% of GP attendees
  • 30% of psychiatric outpatients
  • 40% of psychiatric inpatients.
• People with borderline and (to a lesser extent) antisocial PDs are particularly likely to present to emergency and psychiatric services (because of self-harm and severe emotional reactions to crises).
• Just under half of prisoners have antisocial PD.

Aetiology

Genes and **environment contribute** about equally to personality.
• Genetic influences are shown by twin studies. XYY individuals display higher criminality irrespective of IQ or social class.
• Schizotypal PDs are more common in relatives of people with schizophrenia.
• An underactive autonomic nervous system has been implicated in antisocial PD.

Psychiatry at a Glance, Sixth Edition. Cornelius Katona, Claudia Cooper, Mary Robertson. © 2016 John Wiley & Sons, Ltd. Published 2016 by John Wiley & Sons, Ltd.
Companion website: www.ataglanceseries.com/psychiatry

- Adverse intrauterine, perinatal or postnatal factors leading to abnormal cerebral maturation may predispose to PDs.

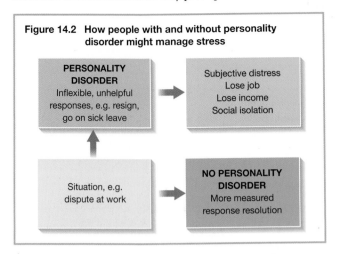

Figure 14.2   How people with and without personality disorder might manage stress

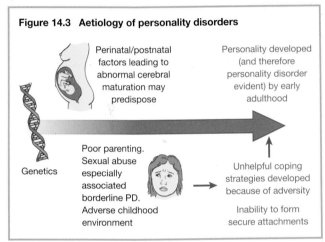

Figure 14.3   Aetiology of personality disorders

- Childhood sexual abuse and borderline PD are strongly linked.
- Poor parenting and an adverse childhood environment (during personality development) are implicated in cognitive and psychodynamic theories.
  - Cognitive theory suggests that people with PDs developed ways of coping with early life adversity (e.g. turning anger against oneself rather than expressing it if this could result in parental violence) that manifest as maladaptive traits later in life (e.g. problems in interpersonal relationships).
  - Psychodynamic theories suggest that PDs result from insecure attachment in childhood and thus in adult relationships.

Classification and characteristics

- Patients (particularly those with severe PDs) often fulfil criteria for more than one PD diagnosis. DSM-5 groups PDs into three clusters that are more likely to overlap. The ICD-10 classification does not include narcissistic PD but is otherwise similar to that of the DSM.
- Figure 14.1 shows the diagnostic criteria.
- People should usually be assessed more than once, collateral history sought and comorbid psychiatric disorders treated before a diagnosis of a PD is made.

Management

- People with PD have in the past been excluded from health and social care, and active work to engage them is needed to reverse

this. Progress is slow but tolerance of frustration is required for effective treatment.
- Structure, consistency and clear boundaries (i.e. agreement of behaviour that is acceptable and unacceptable) are critical. Multidisciplinary and multi-agency work is often required.
- Most people with PDs have a reduced ability to cope with everyday problems, so may need help with housing and other social matters.
- Comorbid psychiatric illness and substance misuse disorders are prevalent, and their detection and treatment are a priority.
- Drugs are sometimes used to treat specific PD traits, e.g. mood stabilisers for impulsivity (not generally recommended because of lack of evidence). Short-term sedative medication may be used cautiously in borderline PD for crisis management.
- Admission to hospital, day hospital care or crisis team input may be necessary during periods of crisis.

The evidence base is strongest for the treatment of antisocial and borderline PD.

Borderline PD

- Adapted cognitive behavioural therapy (CBT), dialectical behaviour therapy (DBT) and mentalisation-based treatments can help (see Chapter 33).
- Threats and acts of deliberate self-harm and suicide can be difficult and time-consuming.
- Ending of or changes in treatments or services may evoke strong emotions and reactions.

Antisocial PD

- Treatment outcomes for antisocial PD are modest, and prevention by targeting children with conduct disorder, a third of whom are likely to develop it, is best (e.g. by providing parent-training/education programmes).
- Psychological therapies require patient cooperation, and motivation to engage in treatment predicts success. For those with a history of offending behaviour, group-based cognitive and behavioural interventions focused on reducing offending and other antisocial behaviour can be effective.
- In the UK there are treatment centres for people with dangerous and severe personality disorders in prisons and secure psychiatric units.

Prognosis

- Most individuals with PDs show decreased aggressive behaviour with age, although the ability to form successful relationships remains poor.
- Borderline PD carries a relatively favourable prognosis with recovery in over 50% at 10–25-year follow-up. It is associated with an increased risk of bipolar affective disorder.
- Schizoid and schizotypal patients tend to remain isolated.
- Dissocial PD carries a particularly poor prognosis.
- Comorbid alcohol and substance misuse is associated with violence and an increased risk of accidental death. There is an increased risk of suicide: 30–60% of completed suicides show evidence of a PD.
- Obsessional PDs are at high risk of progression to obsessive compulsive disorder or depression.
- Paranoid and schizotypal PD may progress to psychosis. Schizoid PD does not predispose to schizophrenia.
- Some PDs may confer susceptibility to physical illness (e.g. obsessional PD and duodenal ulcer).

15 Psychosexual Disorders

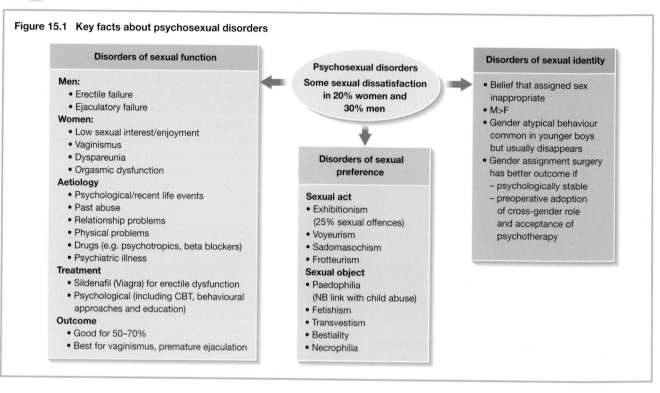

Figure 15.1 Key facts about psychosexual disorders

Disorders of sexual function

Men:
- Erectile failure
- Ejaculatory failure

Women:
- Low sexual interest/enjoyment
- Vaginismus
- Dyspareunia
- Orgasmic dysfunction

Aetiology
- Psychological/recent life events
- Past abuse
- Relationship problems
- Physical problems
- Drugs (e.g. psychotropics, beta blockers)
- Psychiatric illness

Treatment
- Sildenafil (Viagra) for erectile dysfunction
- Psychological (including CBT, behavioural approaches and education)

Outcome
- Good for 50–70%
- Best for vaginismus, premature ejaculation

Psychosexual disorders
Some sexual dissatisfaction in 20% women and 30% men

Disorders of sexual preference

Sexual act
- Exhibitionism (25% sexual offences)
- Voyeurism
- Sadomasochism
- Frotteurism

Sexual object
- Paedophilia (NB link with child abuse)
- Fetishism
- Transvestism
- Bestiality
- Necrophilia

Disorders of sexual identity
- Belief that assigned sex inappropriate
- M>F
- Gender atypical behaviour common in younger boys but usually disappears
- Gender assignment surgery has better outcome if
  – psychologically stable
  – preoperative adoption of cross-gender role and acceptance of psychotherapy

---

- The range of sexual behaviour is extremely wide, with concepts of normality being socially or legally, rather than physiologically, determined.
- Moral and legal objections to some forms of sexual behaviour and an increasing awareness of the seriousness of sexually transmitted infections – particularly the human immunodeficiency virus (HIV) – and of what might be expected from a sexual relationship have encouraged the increasing medicalisation of sexuality.
- Current psychiatric classifications (DSM-5, ICD-10) emphasise that sexual disorders have an element of psychological distress rather than being defined by behaviour alone. They can be divided into disorders of *sexual function*, *preference* and *identity*.

Disorders of sexual function

- Some degree of sexual dissatisfaction is present in as many as 20% of women and 30% of men.
- The commonest problems identified in population surveys and referrals to sexual disorder clinics are:
  - in men: failure of erection and/or ejaculation;
  - in women: low sexual interest, inability to allow penetration (vaginismus), pain on intercourse (dyspareunia), lack of sexual enjoyment and orgasmic dysfunction.
- **Assessment** involves detailed history-taking from, and examination of, both partners in order to identify the nature of the problem, its duration, the couple's knowledge of and attitudes to sex and the reasons why help is currently being sought.

Aetiological factors to be considered in the initial assessment include:
- psychological factors and recent life events;
- past sexual abuse;
- a poor general relationship with the sexual partner;
- physical conditions impeding sexual function, which include:
  - neurological conditions (e.g. multiple sclerosis)
  - diabetes
  - hypothyroidism
  - pelvic surgery;
- sexual dyfunction: this may be a manifestation of poor psychological adjustment to surgery (particularly mastectomy, colostomy or amputation);
- psychiatric conditions:
  - depression (loss of libido, generalised anhedonia)
  - alcohol dependence or misuse
  - anxiety disorders;
- some prescribed drugs including:
  - beta-blockers
  - diuretics
  - antipsychotics
  - benzodiazepines
  - antidepressants
  - recreational drug misuse, especially of opiates.
- **Management** usually involves:
- treatment of underlying medical or psychiatric conditions
- medical treatments:
  - Oral phosphodiesterase inhibitors such as sildenafil (Viagra) are the drugs of choice for erectile dysfunction.

Psychiatry at a Glance, Sixth Edition. Cornelius Katona, Claudia Cooper, Mary Robertson. © 2016 John Wiley & Sons, Ltd. Published 2016 by John Wiley & Sons, Ltd.
Companion website: www.ataglanceseries.com/psychiatry

- Low-dose antidepressant drugs, which have a side effect of delaying time to ejaculation, are also commonly prescribed to men with premature ejaculation.
- Other treatments for erectile dysfunction include mechanical devices (vacuum pumps, penile bands and intracavernosal use of drugs e.g. alprostadil).
- psychological treatments:
  - Cognitive–behavioural-based therapies, which aim to facilitate communication, decrease anxiety about performance failure, and identify and explore underlying developmental and personality problems.
  - Education, particularly dispelling myths about what is considered appropriate or normal sexual behaviour.
  - Traditional sex or couples therapy, which (irrespective of the presenting dysfunction) involves the setting of a hierarchy of sexual 'assignments', structured on behavioural principles.
- **Prognosis** with treatment is good in 50–70% of cases, with best results being for premature ejaculation in men and vaginismus in women. Other favourable prognostic factors include a good quality of general relationship, high motivation and early progress within treatment.

Disorders of sexual preference

Homosexuality is not a disorder of sexual preference. People who are dissatisfied or unhappy with their sexual orientation are almost always so because of disapproval (e.g. of families or religious groups) or discrimination in society.

- Disorders of sexual preference (paraphilias) are much more common in men than in women.
- They may be classified into:
  - variations of the sexual object
  - variations of the sexual act.

Variations of the sexual object include:
- *paedophilia*: sexual activity or fantasy involving children; associated with child pornography and abuse;
- *fetishism*: the object of sexual arousal is an inanimate object (e.g. an item of clothing or a non-genital body part);
- *transvestism*: sexual arousal obtained by cross-dressing;
- *bestiality*: sexual activity with animals;
- *necrophilia*: intercourse with a corpse.

The aetiology of these conditions is unclear.

Management usually involves behaviour therapy (which may involve elements of aversion therapy and conditioning more appropriate responses).

Antiandrogens are sometimes used in paedophilia to help (usually) men reduce or control their sexual desire.

Variations of the sexual act involve the induction of both sexual arousal and (usually) orgasm by specific actions. Almost all people presenting to the courts or for psychiatric treatment with such variations are men. The variations include the following:
- *Exhibitionism* (indecent exposure), which is the most common.
  - Genital exposure is accompanied by emotional tension and excitement and sexual arousal.
  - Exhibitionists make up one-quarter of the sexual offences dealt with by the courts, with psychiatric referral usually arising from this route.
  - Exhibitionists fall into two main groups:
    - those with aggressive personality traits or antisocial personality disorders, in whom the act frequently involves masturbation;
    - those of inhibited temperament, where the exposed penis is often flaccid.
  - Treatment may include psychodynamic, behavioural and hormonal (antiandrogen) components.
- *Voyeurism* (observing sexual acts).
- *Frotteurism* (rubbing the genitalia against a stranger in a crowded place).
- *Sadomasochism* (inflicting pain on others (sadism) or having it inflicted on oneself (masochism)). There are no systematic trials of treatment, although behavioural techniques are often used.

Disorders of sexual identity (*transsexuality*)

- This involves a strong wish to be of the other sex and a conviction that one's biological sex is wrong. Cross-dressing reflects this wish rather than bringing sexual excitement.
- It often begins in childhood, when it is characterised by:
  - cross-dressing,
  - taking cross-gender roles in games and fantasy,
  - an attraction for pastimes usually regarded as more appropriate for children of the opposite sex.
- Gender atypical behaviours in boys are common but they usually disappear because they are discouraged at school and by parents. Most boys who show gender atypical behaviour grow up to be heterosexual although adult homosexual men are more likely to report gender atypical behaviour in childhood than are heterosexual men.
- Boys with clinical disorders of sexual identity do not regard themselves as homosexual as they grow up but rather as a woman (in a man's body) who is attracted to men.
- Most adult transsexuals are men. Transsexuals usually seek gender-reassignment surgery (with associated hormonal treatment). Outcome following such treatment is best where the patient:
  - is psychologically stable,
  - has adopted the cross-gender role consistently for at least two years prior to surgery,
  - accepts that surgical treatment is not a 'cure',
  - is willing to participate in presurgical psychotherapy.

16 Unusual Psychiatric Syndromes

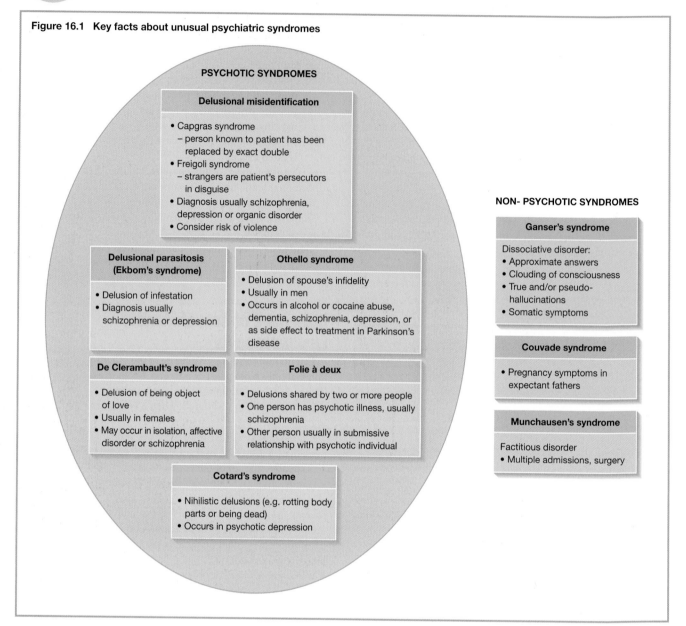

Figure 16.1 Key facts about unusual psychiatric syndromes

PSYCHOTIC SYNDROMES

Delusional misidentification

- Capgras syndrome
  - person known to patient has been replaced by exact double
- Freigoli syndrome
  - strangers are patient's persecutors in disguise
- Diagnosis usually schizophrenia, depression or organic disorder
- Consider risk of violence

Delusional parasitosis (Ekbom's syndrome)

- Delusion of infestation
- Diagnosis usually schizophrenia or depression

Othello syndrome

- Delusion of spouse's infidelity
- Usually in men
- Occurs in alcohol or cocaine abuse, dementia, schizophrenia, depression, or as side effect to treatment in Parkinson's disease

De Clerambault's syndrome

- Delusion of being object of love
- Usually in females
- May occur in isolation, affective disorder or schizophrenia

Folie à deux

- Delusions shared by two or more people
- One person has psychotic illness, usually schizophrenia
- Other person usually in submissive relationship with psychotic individual

Cotard's syndrome

- Nihilistic delusions (e.g. rotting body parts or being dead)
- Occurs in psychotic depression

NON- PSYCHOTIC SYNDROMES

Ganser's syndrome

Dissociative disorder:
- Approximate answers
- Clouding of consciousness
- True and/or pseudo-hallucinations
- Somatic symptoms

Couvade syndrome

- Pregnancy symptoms in expectant fathers

Munchausen's syndrome

Factitious disorder
- Multiple admissions, surgery

- The features of the best described psychiatric syndromes are summarised below.
- Although these syndromes have now been subsumed into the ICD-10 and DSM-5 classification systems, their names are still in regular use.
- They can be divided into psychotic (characterised by delusions and hallucinations) and non-psychotic syndromes.

Psychotic syndromes
Delusional misidentification syndrome

- The two most common subtypes are:
  - Capgras' syndrome, characterised by a delusional belief that a person known to the patient (e.g. spouse or parent) has been replaced by an imposter who is their exact double;

- Fregoli's syndrome, which involves the delusion that strangers or other people the patient meets (e.g. nurses, doctors) are the patient's persecutors in disguise.
- It most commonly occurs in schizophrenia, affective disorders and dementia or other organic illness. Treatment is of the primary disorder.
- There is some evidence that it relates to the pathophysiology of face recognition, with hyporecognition in Capgras' and hyperrecognition in Fregoli's syndrome.
- Violence towards those who are the subject of the delusions is rare but the risk should be assessed carefully.

Delusional parasitosis

- This is also known as Ekbom's syndrome (although this term is also used to describe the neurological disorder of 'restless legs').

Psychiatry at a Glance, Sixth Edition. Cornelius Katona, Claudia Cooper, Mary Robertson. © 2016 John Wiley & Sons, Ltd. Published 2016 by John Wiley & Sons, Ltd.
Companion website: www.ataglanceseries.com/psychiatry

- It is twice as common in women.
- Sufferers believe that insects are colonising their body, particularly the skin and eyes. They often claim to feel dermal sensations and to visualise the bugs, although no one else can see them.
- Initial presentation is often to public health workers (with persistent demands for deinfestation), dermatologists or infectious disease physicians, with insistent, repeated and bizarre requests for investigation and treatment.
- Delusions may be circumscribed or part of a schizophrenic or depressive illness.
- Antipsychotics are the mainstay of treatment.

Folie à deux (induced or shared delusional disorder)

- A delusional belief that is shared by two or more people (usually within a family), of whom only one has a psychotic illness.
- The psychotic individual (principal) tends to be more intelligent and better educated than the non-psychotic (more submissive) recipient(s) and has a dominating influence over them.
- The delusion is usually persecutory or hypochondriacal.
- The pair are often isolated from others by distance or by cultural or language barriers.
- The diagnosis of the principal is most commonly schizophrenia but may be an affective disorder or dementia.
- Folie à deux is classified as induced delusional disorder in ICD-10; DSM-5 does not list it separately from delusional disorder.
- Primary treatment of the principal is of the underlying condition. A period of separation of the involved individuals, followed by supportive individual and/or family therapy, may be helpful.

De Clerambault's syndrome (erotomania)

- The patient (usually female) has the unfounded and delusional belief that someone (usually a man of higher social status) is in love with her. The patient makes inappropriate advances to this person and becomes angry (and sometimes violent) when rejected.
- The syndrome may exist in isolation, as part of an affective (usually manic) disorder or, more rarely, schizophrenia.
- Underlying conditions should be treated; where no other underlying condition is identified, antipsychotics may be useful.
- Management frequently involves hospitalisation (sometimes compulsory) to prevent harassment or injury. When men are affected they present a greater forensic risk.

Othello syndrome (morbid or pathological jealousy)

- The patient (usually male) is delusionally convinced that his partner is being unfaithful. He goes to great lengths to produce 'evidence' of the infidelity (e.g. stains on underclothes/sheets) and to extract a confession.
- It may occur in long-term alcohol abuse, dementia, schizophrenia, cocaine addiction and as a side effect of treatment with dopamine agonists in Parkinson's disease.
- Paradoxically, the partner is sometimes driven to true and actual infidelity.
- There is a substantial risk of violence (even homicide); thus, distant separation may be warranted and compulsory hospitalisation and treatment are often necessary. It tends to reoccur with a new partner.

Cotard's syndrome

- This is characterised by nihilistic delusions in which the patient believes that parts of his or her body are decaying or rotting or have ceased to exist. Patients may also believe themselves to be dead or (paradoxically) unable to die and therefore eternally alive.
- It is almost invariably found in the context of psychotic depression.
- Electroconvulsive therapy (ECT) is often required because of the severity of the associated depression.

Non-psychotic syndromes
Munchausen's syndrome

- Munchausen's syndrome is termed 'factitious disorder' in ICD-10 and DSM-5.
- It is characterised by deliberately feigned symptomatology, usually physical (e.g. abdominal pain) but sometimes psychiatric (e.g. with feigned hallucinations, multiple bereavements or sexual abuse).
- These result in multiple presentations to A&E departments, usually to several hospitals, with frequent admissions often culminating in surgical procedures.
- Patients often use multiple aliases, are often of no fixed abode and usually have no regular GP. When discovered, the patients usually discharge themselves against medical advice.
- The syndrome characteristically occurs in people with severe personality disorders.
- Management is difficult, although confrontation without rejection may prove helpful.
- Important differential diagnoses are dissociative and somatisation disorders (where symptoms are not consciously produced) and undiagnosed illness.
- Occasionally the disorder can be by proxy, as when a parent fakes illnesses in a child (***Munchausen's syndrome by proxy***).

Couvade syndrome

- This is the experience of symptoms resembling those of pregnancy (abdominal swelling and/or spasms, nausea and vomiting, etc.) in expectant fathers. Anxiety and psychosomatic symptoms (e.g. toothache) are also common.
- The prevalence of mild forms is as high as 20%.
- The condition (which in some cultures is quite acceptable and may even be expected) is usually self-limiting and responds to counselling but often recurs in subsequent pregnancies.

Ganser's syndrome

- This is a rare, dissociative disorder (Chapter 27). Symptoms are seen as a defence against intolerable stress.
- Characteristic symptoms are:
  - approximate, absurd and often inconsistent answers to simple questions. The patient may say '2 + 2 = 5', or, when asked the colour of snow, reply 'green';
  - clouding of consciousness;
  - true and/or pseudohallucinations (visual or auditory);
  - somatic symptoms.
- There may be an underlying depressive illness warranting treatment in its own right.
- It is overrepresented in prison populations.
- Spontaneous improvement often occurs and is characteristically accompanied by amnesia for the abnormal behaviour. Recovery may be hastened by admission to hospital and psychotherapeutic exploration of underlying conflicts.
- Factitious disorder is a differential diagnosis.

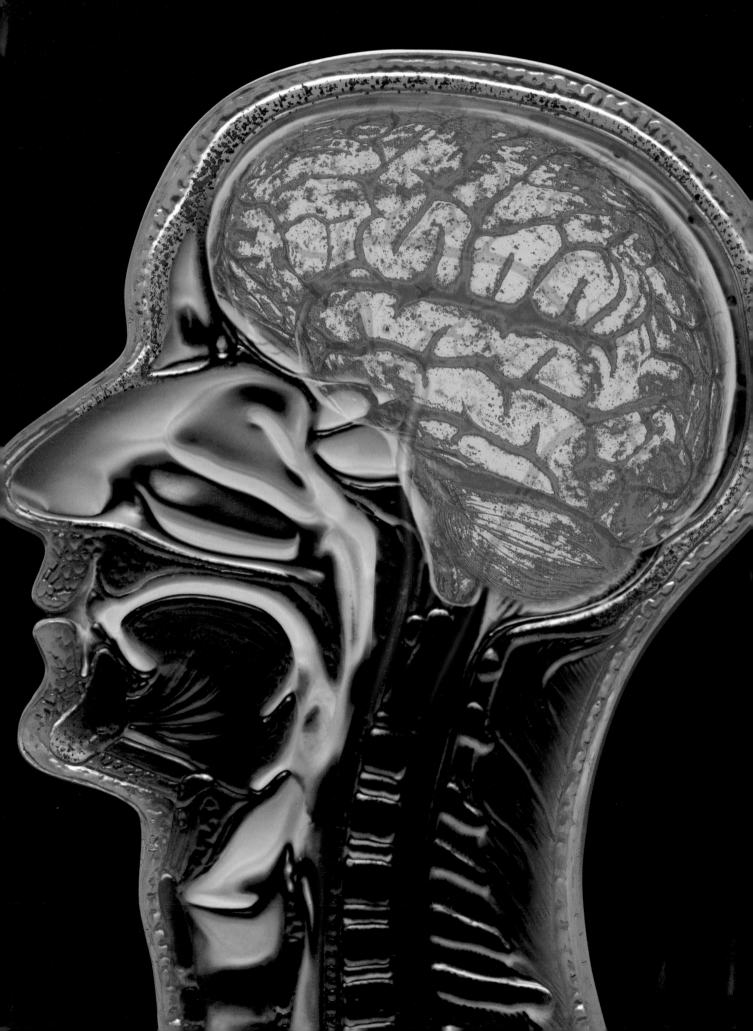

Substance and Alcohol Misuse

Part 3

Chapters

17 Substance Misuse

Figure 17.1 Key facts about substances and their misuse

	OPIATES	STIMULANTS	HALLUCINOGENS	CANNABIS
Includes	• Heroin • Morphine • Methadone	• Cocaine • Amphetamines	• Ecstasy (MDMA), • Gammahydroxybutyrate (GHB) • Gamma-butyrolactone (GBL) • LSD, magic mushrooms	Active compound is tetrahydrocannabinol
Taken	Smoked, snorted, oral, iv, subcutaneously	Snorted, iv.	Oral	Smoked, oral
Effect	Intensely pleasurable buzz or rush→peace, detachment→central nervous system depression	Brief high with euphoria, ▲energy and concentration	• Stimulant • Hallucinogenic	• Euphoria, relaxation, • Hallucinations • ▲appetite and ▼body temperature
Negative effect	• Signs of dependence: miosis, tremor, malaise, apathy, constipation, weakness, impotence, neglect, malnutrition • 2–3% dependent users die annually • iv. use can lead to HIV, hepatitis B, C • Overdose: miosis, respiratory depression, death	• Depression/tiredness follow use • Psychosis	• Ecstasy, GHB, GBL: Potentially fatal dehydration/hyponatraemia from excess water consumption • LSD: rarely flashbacks/psychosis and (in overdose) seizures	• Conjunctival irritation ▼spermatogenesis • Lung disease • Flashbacks, transient psychosis, schizophrenia • Depression, apathy
Dependence	• 10% of users physically dependent • Tolerance and withdrawal develop quickly	Psychological dependence common		
Management	• Residential or community • Methadone or buprenorphine, for detox or maintenance • Contingency management • Harm reduction (e.g. needle exchange)	Usually community psychological therapy can help		

Epidemiology

• One in 10 UK adults and 17% of those aged 11–15 have used illicit drugs. There is a strong association with younger age (11–24 years) and male gender.
• Between 3 and 4% of teenagers and adults have used class A drugs in the last year.
• Cannabis is the most common illicit drug used, followed by cocaine, ecstasy, amphetamines and amyl nitrate.

Classification

ICD-10 classifies substance use disorders according to (1) substance and (2) type of disorder. The latter include the following:

Acute intoxication: transient disturbances of consciousness, cognition, perception, affect or behaviour following the administration of a psychoactive substance (PS).

Harmful use: damage to the individual's health and adverse effects on family and society.

Dependence: Figure 17.2 shows the signs of dependence. There is usually an associated neglect of important social, occupational or recreational activities.

Withdrawal state: physical and psychological symptoms occurring on absolute or relative withdrawal of a substance after repeated, usually prolonged and/or high-dose use.

Psychotic disorder: psychosis during or immediately after use, with vivid hallucinations, abnormal affect, psychomotor disturbances and delusions of persecution and reference.

Amnesic disorder: memory and other cognitive impairments caused by substance use (e.g. alcohol, see Chapter 18).

Figure 17.2 Signs of dependence

Compulsion to take substance **S**topping causes withdrawal
Aware of harms but persist **T**ime preoccupied with substance ▲
N'eglect of other activities **O**ut of control of use
Tolerance **P**ersistent, futile wish to cut down

Residual and late onset psychotic disorders: effects on behaviour, affect, personality or cognition that last beyond the period during which a direct PS effect might be expected (e.g. flashbacks).

Aetiological factors

• Availability and peer pressure.
• Desire for pleasurable effects. All drugs of abuse activate the dopamine system in the mesolimbic reward pathway.
• Prescribed drugs may be misused.
• Psychiatric illness:
  • Impulsivity or anxiety may increase drug use.
  • Patients with borderline and antisocial personality disorders are much more likely to take illicit drugs.
  • Conversely, substance misuse can exacerbate low mood and anxiety, or precipitate psychosis.
  • Management of patients with psychiatric and coexisting substance use disorders (dual diagnosis) should optimally involve a multidisciplinary team trained to manage both disorders.

Psychiatry at a Glance, Sixth Edition. Cornelius Katona, Claudia Cooper, Mary Robertson. © 2016 John Wiley & Sons, Ltd. Published 2016 by John Wiley & Sons, Ltd.
Companion website: www.ataglanceseries.com/psychiatry

Figure 17.3 Aetiology of substance misuse

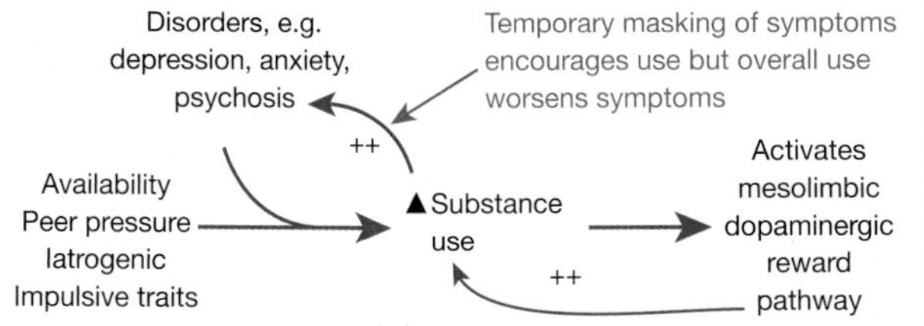

Figure 17.4 Substance misuse and the UK law

Drugs can be legally acquired from chemists (codeine), shops (solvents) or doctors (benzodiazepines, opiates). The UK Misuse of Drugs Act controls and classifies illicit drugs:

Class A – opiates, hallucinogens, injected stimulants
Class B – cannabis and amphetamines
Class C – ketamine and GHB (gamma-hydroxybutyric acid)

More harmful
Harsher penalties

Unclassified drugs include amyl nitrite (poppers) and 'legal highs' (psychoactive substances manufactured to try to escape legal sanctions)

Management

- Can be in residential rehabilitation, hospital or community.
- Contingency management programmes are evidence based. Drug users receiving methadone or who misuse stimulants are offered rewards (e.g. vouchers for goods or services) for negative drug tests or harm reduction (e.g. hepatitis and HIV tests).
- Effective psychosocial interventions include cognitive behavioural therapy, motivational interviewing (see Chapter 18) and self-help groups.
- Medication can be useful (see specific substances below).
- Infection (HIV and hepatitis C) is the greatest risk associated with injecting drug use; harm-reduction strategies aim to minimise infection (e.g. needle exchange) and improve safety.

Specific substances

Opiates

- Figure 17.1 lists the opiates of abuse and their effects.
- Ten per cent of opiate misusers become dependent, but only 10% of these ever seek help; 2–3% die annually. Of the remainder, 25% are abstinent at five years and 40% at 10 years.
- Tolerance and withdrawal develop quickly. Early withdrawal symptoms (24–48 hours) include craving, flu-like symptoms, sweating and yawning. Mydriasis (dilation of the pupil), abdominal cramps, diarrhoea, agitation, restlessness, piloerection ('gooseflesh') and tachycardia occur later (7–10 days).
- Opiate detoxification treatment usually lasts 4–12 weeks:
  - **Methadone** (opioid agonist) or **buprenorphine** (opioid partial agonist) are first line; they are less euphoriant and have a relatively long half-life than opioids of abuse.
  - **Lofexidine** is sometimes used for short detoxification treatments or where abuse is mild or uncertain.
  - Consider a contingency management programme, with psychosocial support for at least six months.
- In maintenance therapy, methadone or buprenorphine is prescribed at a dose higher than required to prevent withdrawal symptoms. This can reduce craving, prevent withdrawal, eliminate the hazards of injecting and stop illicit drug use. The aim is progression from maintenance to detoxification and abstinence.
- **Naltrexone** (opioid antagonist) blocks the euphoric effects and is occasionally used to help prevent relapse.
- Signs of overdose (often accidental) include miosis and respiratory depression and may require **naloxone**.

Hallucinogens

- See Figure 17.1. Magic mushrooms have similar but less prolonged effects to LSD.

Stimulants

- *Cocaine* may be sniffed, chewed or injected intravenously.
  - Its effects (restlessness, increased energy, abolition of fatigue and hunger) resemble hypomania and last about 20 minutes. Visual/tactile hallucinations of insects (formication) and paranoid psychoses occur.
  - Post-cocaine dysphoria, with sleeplessness and intense depression, precedes withdrawal (depression, insomnia and craving).
  - 'Crack' (a purified, very addictive form of cocaine) is smoked. The crack 'high' is extremely short and, on withdrawal, persecutory delusions are common.
- *Amphetamines* ('speed'), taken orally or intravenously, cause euphoria, increased concentration and energy, mydriasis, tachycardia and hyperreflexia, followed by depression, fatigue and headache. Acute use may cause psychosis.
- *Methamphetamine* is chemically related but more potent, longlasting and harmful; it can be ingested, snorted or smoked (as crystal meth).
- *Naphyrone* and *mephedrone* are also closely related to amphetamines. They were originally manufactured as 'legal highs' (see box) but are now class B drugs.
- *Amyl nitrite* and butyl nitrite and isobutyl nitrite (called 'poppers') are sniffed from small bottles. They deliver a short, sharp high. Side effects include severe headache and feeling faint. They are toxic and can be fatal if swallowed.

Other drugs

- *Cannabis*: see Figure 17.1.
- *Benzodiazepines* produce dependence, withdrawal (including seizures) and tolerance. Dependence is often iatrogenic, although benzodiazepines are also common street drugs.
- *Solvents*
  - Typically sniffed, principally by boys (aged 8–19 years) (a red rash around the mouth and nose may be a sign of abuse).
  - Initial euphoria is followed by drowsiness.
  - Psychological dependence is common but physical dependence is rare.
  - Chronic abuse results in weight loss, nausea, vomiting, polyneuropathy and cognitive impairment.
  - Toxic effects (can be fatal): bronchospasm, arrythmias, aplastic anaemia, hepatorenal and cerebral damage.
- *Phencyclidine* (PCP; 'Angel Dust') is usually smoked. Its effects include euphoria, peripheral analgesia and impaired consciousness or psychosis, which may require antipsychotics.
- *Khat*:
  - used particularly by men from Somalia and Yemen;
  - contains cathinone, an amphetamine-like stimulant causing excitement and euphoria;
  - not a controlled substance in the UK.

18 Alcohol Misuse

Alcohol abuse is regular or binge consumption of alcohol sufficient to cause physical, neuropsychiatric or social damage.

Safe limits

- A 'unit' of alcohol (10 mL, 8 g) is roughly a small glass of wine, a pub single of spirits or a half pint of beer.
- The conventional safe drinking limits are 21 units per week for men and 14 for women, with at least two drink-free days each week.
- The UK government gives guidelines for maximum daily use (<4 units a day for men, <3 units for women), reflecting concerns about binge-drinking.
- Much smaller amounts may be hazardous to a foetus.

Classification

ICD-10 classifies alcohol use disorders using the same system as for other psychoactive substances (see Chapter 17).

- **Acute intoxication** is characterised by slurred speech, impaired coordination and judgement, labile affect and, in severe cases, hypoglycaemia, stupor and coma. Differential diagnosis includes other causes of acute confusion, particularly head trauma.
- **Acute withdrawal** reflects the degree of previous dependence and usually occurs within one to two days of abstinence.
  - It is characterised by malaise, nausea, autonomic hyperactivity, tremulousness, labile mood, insomnia and transient hallucinations or illusions (usually visual).
  - Seizures are a recognised complication.
  - Severe withdrawal, or 'delirium tremens' ('shaking delirium'), occurs in 5% of withdrawals and has a mortality of up to 15%, partly as a result of other medical complications.
- **Alcohol dependence**:

Figure 18.1 Signs of alcohol dependence

Compulsion/strong desire to drink alcohol

Aware of physical/psychological harms but persist

N'eglect of other activities

Tolerance to alcohol

Stopping causes withdrawal

Stereotyped pattern of drinking

Time preoccupied with alcohol ▲

Out of control of use

Persistent, futile wish to cut down

- **Psychotic disorders** related to alcohol use include:
  - alcoholic hallucinosis (usually threatening, second-person voices in a clear sensorium)
  - jealousy (paranoid delusions about infidelity).
- **Amnesic disorder**: for example, Korsakoff's psychosis (see glossary).
- **Residual and late onset disorders**: include depression and dementia.

Epidemiology

- Prevalence rates worldwide vary widely and are related to overall consumption levels, availability and price.

- In the UK, heavy drinking (an average of 8 units/day for men and 6 units/day for women) is reported by 23% of men and 9% of women; younger people are more likely to exceed safe limits.
- The prevalence of alcohol dependence is 6% in men and 2% in women. Rates are particularly high in medical inpatients and are increasing in women and adolescents.
- Alcohol abuse and dependence often begin in the early to mid-20s, at a time when most people begin to moderate their drinking as their responsibilities increase.

Detection and screening

- A fifth of primary care attenders have an alcohol use disorder.
- The detection of disorders can be difficult because they are not usually clinically obvious, but is crucial to:
  - enable appropriate treatment
  - avoid long-term complications
  - avoid withdrawal from unplanned abstinence (e.g. after surgery).
- Professionals should have a high index of suspicion in medical inpatients and those with mental illness or two or more drink-driving offences.
- Many cases can be detected by documenting a typical drinking week.
- Screening questionnaires are also helpful:

Fig. 18.2 Screening tests.

The CAGE questionnaire

Have you tried to **C**ut down drinking?
Have people **A**nnoyed you by suggesting you do so?
Have you felt **G**uilty about drinking?
Have you needed an **E**ye-opener (early morning drink)?

Fast Alcohol Scoring Test (FAST)

	Question		Score
1. >8 drinks (men) >6 drinks women	1–3	Never	0
(Continue if score ≥1)		<monthly	1
		Monthly	2
2. Can't remember the night before		Weekly	3
3. Failed to function normally because of alcohol		Daily	4
4. Someone else is concerned about your drinking	4	No	0
		Once	1
Score of 2 or more = hazardous drinking		>once	2

- Collateral history can be revealing.
- Physical examination may reveal alcoholic stigmata, particularly signs of liver disease (jaundice, spider naevi, palmar erythema, gynaecomastia) and peripheral neuropathy.
- Macrocytosis without anaemia and raised γ-glutamyl transferase (GGT), alanine and aspartate aminotransferase (ALT and AST) or carbohydrate deficient transferrin (CDT) indicate recent harmful use.

Aetiology

This is multifactorial. Factors include the following:
- A strong genetic component (around 60%), which appears to be multigenic. Genetically determined alterations in alcohol

Psychiatry at a Glance, Sixth Edition. Cornelius Katona, Claudia Cooper, Mary Robertson. © 2016 John Wiley & Sons, Ltd. Published 2016 by John Wiley & Sons, Ltd.
Companion website: www.ataglanceseries.com/psychiatry

metabolism may partially explain this, with those at low risk producing more (hangover-causing) acetaldehyde; 50% of Japanese people have an unpleasant 'flush reaction' on drinking alcohol due to a mutation in the acetaldehyde dehydrogenase 2 gene. There is often a positive family history of depression.

• Occupation: high-risk groups include the armed forces, doctors, publicans, journalists.

• Cultural influences: low rates are reported in Jews and Muslims, and high rates in Scottish and Irish people.

• The cost of alcoholic drinks.

• Behavioural models stress:
  • learning by imitation (modelling)
  • social reinforcement
  • the association between drinking and pleasure (classical conditioning)
  • avoiding withdrawal symptoms (operant conditioning).

• Risk increases in the presence of chronic psychiatric or physical illness, particularly if complicated by chronic pain. There is an association with mood and anxiety disorders.

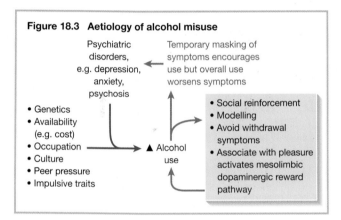

Figure 18.3 Aetiology of alcohol misuse

Complications

• *Neuropsychiatric complications*:
  • Wernicke's encephalopathy:

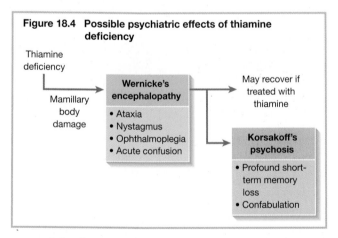

Figure 18.4 Possible psychiatric effects of thiamine deficiency

  • peripheral neuropathy
  • erectile or ejaculatory impotence
  • cerebellar degeneration
  • dementia.

• *Other physical complications*: drinking damages almost every organ system in the body.

• *Social complications* include unemployment, marital difficulties, criminality, prostitution, homicides, domestic violence, accidental deaths, road accidents and suicides.

• *Psychiatric complications*:
Repeated heavy drinking is associated with:
  • a 40% risk of temporary depressive episodes
  • suicidal ideas and attempts
  • severe anxiety
  • insomnia.
These often improve within two to four weeks of abstinence.

• *Foetal alcohol syndrome* (from drinking in pregnancy) is characterised by:
  • decreased muscle tone
  • poor coordination
  • developmental delay
  • heart defects
  • a range of facial abnormalities.

Management

• Abstinence is the usual goal for treatment of dependence, although sometimes it is controlled drinking.

• Achieving abstinence requires *acute detoxification*:
  • This should be in hospital if there is a risk of delirium tremens or withdrawal seizures, or the person is a child or vulnerable (e.g. cognitively impaired or lacking support).
  • Initially high but rapidly tailing sedation (almost always a benzodiazepine, such as chlordiazepoxide or diazepam) is usually needed to control withdrawal symptoms and prevent seizures.
  • Treatment of delirium tremens is usually with lorazepam or antipsychotics (e.g. haloperidol or olanzapine).
  • Treatment also includes rehydration, correction of electrolyte disturbance, and oral or parenteral thiamine.

• *Motivational interviewing* is client-centred counselling that explores ambivalence to seeking treatment, drinking cessation or both. It may help problem drinkers in denial achieve insight and a desire to change.

• *Psychological therapies* (individually or in groups) may promote maintenance of abstinence or controlled drinking (i.e. within safe limits). They are useful for:
  • sustaining motivation
  • learning relapse-prevention strategies
  • developing social routines not reliant on alcohol
  • treating coexistent depression and anxiety.

• *Self-help groups* (e.g. Alcoholics Anonymous) are effective; they reduce pro-drinking activities and social ties.

• *Medication* may help maintain abstinence after detoxification:
  • Disulfiram blocks alcohol metabolism, inducing acetaldehyde accumulation if alcohol is ingested, with resultant flushing, headache, anxiety and nausea.
  • Acamprosate acts on the γ-aminobutyric acid (GABA) system to reduce cravings and risk of relapse.
  • Naltrexone, an opioid-receptor antagonist, has similar therapeutic effects.

• *Prevention measures* include:
  • increasing taxation on alcohol
  • restricting its advertising or sale
  • school alcohol education: this reduces long-term alcohol use, risky alcohol-related behaviour and binge-drinking.

Prognosis

• Continued alcohol problems increase the rate of early death by a factor of three or four. The most common causes are heart disease, stroke, cancers, liver cirrhosis, accidents and suicide.

• Only 15% of those with alcohol use disorder seek treatment; those who do have a better prognosis.

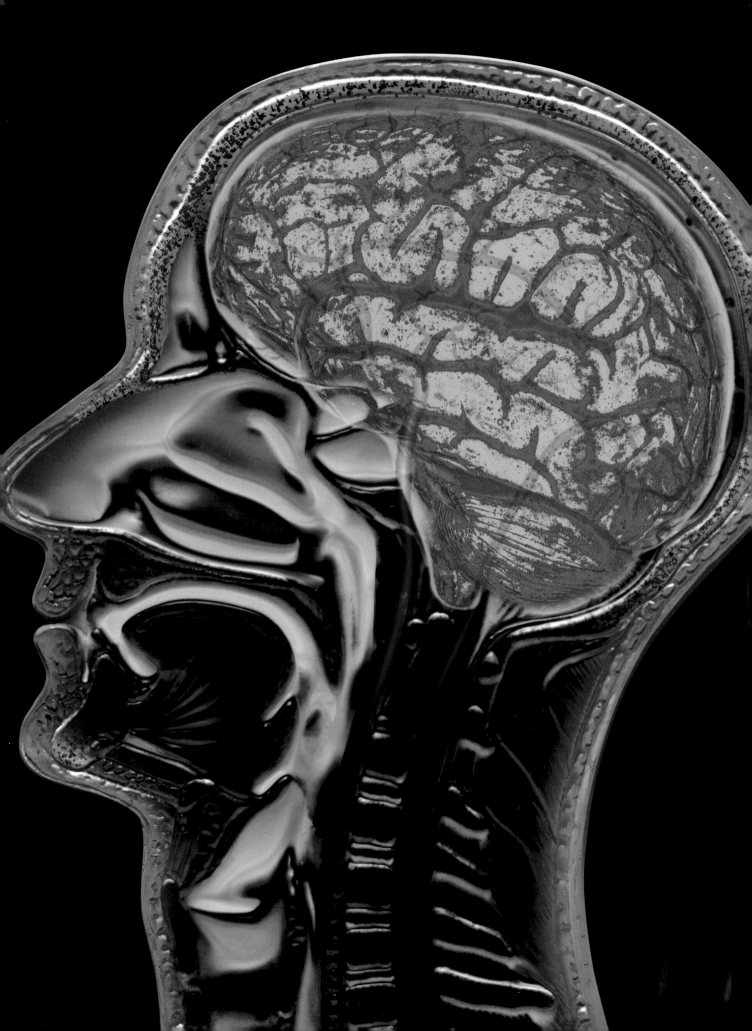

Psychiatry of Demographic Groups

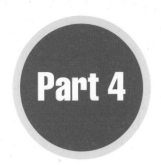

Part 4

Chapters

19 Child Psychiatry I

Classification

- Figure 19.1 shows how ICD-10 classifies childhood psychiatric disorders. DSM-5 categorises ADHD, autistic spectrum and communication disorders, intellectual disability (Chapter 22), specific learning and motor disorders including Tourette's disorder as neurodevelopmental disorders. Emotional and conduct disorders are categorised with adult disorders of emotion (depression/anxiety) and conduct/personality (Chapter 3).

Psychiatric assessment of children

Interview the child, parental figures and teachers. Ask about:
- current behavioural or emotional difficulties (including mood, sleep, appetite, elimination, relationships and antisocial behaviours);
- school behaviour and academic performance;
- daily routine (including hobbies);
- family structure and interactions and past or current separations.

Look for signs of abuse or neglect (Figure 19.2), interaction with parental figures and parenting style. Physical, including neurological, examination is an important part of the assessment.

Epidemiology

- About 10% of boys and 6% of girls aged 5–10 years have an emotional or behavioural disorder, with the excess in boys due to higher rates of hyperkinetic ADHD and conduct disorders.
- Figure 19.3 shows the main childhood disorders and their relationship to gender and age.

Hyperkinetic disorders (ICD-10); Attention-Deficit Hyperactivity Disorder (ADHD) (DSM-5)

- Core symptoms are the presence for at least six months of:
  - short attention span
  - distractibility
  - overactivity
  - impulsivity.
- Symptoms are almost always present by the age of 7, and occur in at least two settings (e.g. home and school).
- It is less commonly recognised in the UK (using ICD-10 criteria) (<1%) than in the USA (7%) (using DSM-5 criteria), probably reflecting the UK's narrower concept of ADHD.
- ADHD frequently coexists with:
  - conduct disorder
  - anxiety and/or depression
  - language delay
  - specific reading retardation
  - antisocial behaviour
  - clumsiness.
- Comorbidity predicts a poorer prognosis. Children with comorbid ADHD and conduct disorder are at particular risk of substance misuse disorders in adolescence.

Figure 19.1 ICD-10 classification of childhood psychiatric disorders

Disorders specific to childhood

Behavioural and emotional disorders
- Hyperkinetic disorders (ADHD)
- Conduct disorders
  - unsocialised
  - socialised
  - oppositional defiant disorder
- Emotional disorders
  - separation anxiety disorder
  - social anxiety disorder
  - sibling rivalry disorder
- Social functioning disorders
  - elective mutism
  - reactive attachment disorder
- Other disorders
  - enuresis
  - encopresis

Disorders of psychological development
- Pervasive developmental disorders
  - autism/autistic spectrum disorder (ASD)
  - Asperger's syndrome
  - childhood disintegrative disorder
- Specific developmental disorders e.g. specific reading retardation

Disorders with onset in childhood or adulthood

- Depression
- Anxiety disorders
  - phobias
  - OCD
- Adjustment disorders
  - bereavement
- Psychotic disorders
- Sleep problems

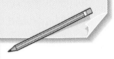

Figure 19.2 Child abuse (physical, emotional, sexual) and neglect

Aetiology	Signs
Child • Low birthweight • Intellectual or physical impairment • Persistently restless or crying **Parents** • Young/single • Disadvantaged • Isolated • Own history of abuse • Didn't want child • Unrealistic discipline	**Physical** • Unexplained injuries **Sexual** • Age inappropriate sexual talk, behaviour or play • Secondary enuresis • Sexually transmitted infections • Nightmares **Any** • Withdrawn/fearful of parents • Failure to thrive
Effects	**What to do?**
Childhood • Emotional disorders, conduct disorders, developmental disorders **Adulthood** • Depression, personality disorders, conversion disorders (e.g. pseudoseizures) • Deliberate self-harm • Child-rearing problems	• Report suspicions, in UK to social services • Involve police if needed • Individual or family therapy

Psychiatry at a Glance, Sixth Edition. Cornelius Katona, Claudia Cooper, Mary Robertson. © 2016 John Wiley & Sons, Ltd. Published 2016 by John Wiley & Sons, Ltd.
Companion website: www.ataglanceseries.com/psychiatry

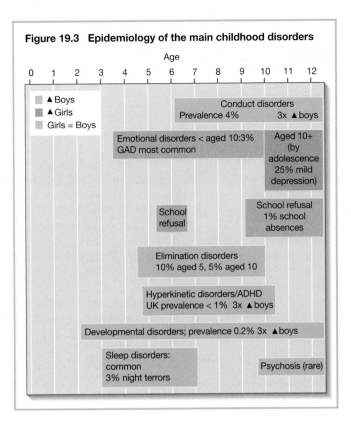

Figure 19.3 Epidemiology of the main childhood disorders

- Aetiological factors include:
  - genetic loading
  - social adversity
  - parental alcohol abuse
  - dietary constituents (lead, tartrazine)
  - exposure to tranquillisers.

Severe forms are often associated with low intelligence, particularly in the context of brain damage (cerebral palsy, epilepsy).

- Treatment approaches include:
  - parent training/education programmes;
  - classroom behavioural interventions by trained teachers;
  - methylphenidate in school-age children;
  - sometimes atomoxetine, a noradrenaline reuptake inhibitor.
- In the majority of patients, the ADHD continues into adulthood, but diagnosis is frequently not made, they are not treated, and there are numerous adverse consequences including an excess of adult antisocial behaviour. Hyperactivity usually lessens by adolescence but learning difficulties may persist.

Conduct disorders

- These are characterised by persistent disruptive, deceptive and aggressive behaviours, including:

disobedience	damage to property
truancy	lying
stealing	fighting
use of force and weapons	arson

- The prevalence (4%) is higher in lower social classes.
- Conduct disorders are associated with:
  - low self-esteem (poor peer relationships in 20%)
  - hyperkinetic disorders ADHD
  - learning or developmental disorders.

- They are categorised as:
  - *socialised* conduct disorder – where behaviours are viewed as normal within the peer group or family;
  - *unsocialised* conduct disorder – where behaviours are solitary, with peer and parental rejection.
- Aetiological factors include:
  - family disharmony;
  - harsh, violent, inconsistent parenting;
  - parents with alcohol dependence, antisocial personality disorder or depression.
- Management involves sessions (typically 8–12) of group or individual parent-training/education programmes. These aim to:
  - help parents understand their own and their child's emotions and behaviour;
  - improve parents' communication with their child;
  - use behavioural management principles (Chapter 33) to help parents improve their child's problem behaviours, e.g. through role-play, and homework to use rehearsed behaviours at home.
- Cognitive–behavioural and social skills therapies may target the child's aggressive behaviour or poor social interactions.
- Antisocial behaviours persist into adult life in two-thirds of children with conduct disorder. Adults with antisocial personality disorder, substance, affective, anxiety and eating disorders, schizophrenia and mania, are more likely to have had conduct disorder.
- **Oppositional defiant disorder** is:
  - usually seen in children under the age of 10 years;
  - characterised by persistent, angry and defiant behaviours;
  - similar to conduct disorder without severe aggressive or dissocial acts, and has a better prognosis.

Emotional disorders

- As well as anxiety and depressive disorders, which occur in all ages, ICD-10 includes diagnoses describing unusually severe or persistent emotional responses to normal developmental phases (e.g. *separation anxiety disorder* and *sibling rivalry disorder*). Treatment involves behavioural and family therapy.

- *Generalised anxiety*, the most common emotional disorder in childhood, has autonomic (palpitations, dry mouth) and psychological (fear) components. Somatic symptoms, particularly abdominal pain, are common. Predisposing factors include the child's temperament and parental overprotection.

- *Phobias*, particularly of the dark or of strangers, are common in small children and usually not clinically significant. When persistent and intense (often in response to parental or social reinforcement) the avoidance may become pathological.

- *Depression* presents similarly to the adult disorder. Treatment involves psychological therapies. Current UK guidelines do not recommend the routine use of antidepressants (see Chapter 8); selective serotonin reuptake inhibitors (SSRIs) have been linked to suicidal or aggressive behaviour (fluoxetine is an exception, although careful monitoring is still advised).

- Completed suicide is rare in children, and equally prevalent in boys and girls. Attempted suicide is more common in girls (3× boys) and lower social classes.

- *Bereavement reactions* are common, with similar symptoms and stages of grief to adults. They may last for several months. Enuresis and temper tantrums in younger children, and sleep disturbance, poor school performance, acting-out behaviours and depressive illness in older children, may ensue. Where a parent has died, the surviving parent's coping mechanisms are crucial.

- *Obsessive–compulsive disorder* (OCD). Isolated obsessions and compulsions (e.g. not walking on paving-stone lines) are common in childhood. The prevalence of OCD is estimated to be around 0.3–1%. OCD presents much as in adults and usually responds to cognitive behavioural therapy (usually requiring family cooperation). Fluoxetine may be prescribed cautiously.

- *School refusal* is not a diagnosis in itself. Child anxiety, bullying and difficult family dynamics are common causes. It accounts for 1% of school absences, with no gender or social class differences. It may present with somatic symptoms (headache, abdominal pain). Three peak ages are recognised: aged 5–6 years (separation anxiety); aged 10–11 years (school transition); and adolescents (12+ years) (low self-esteem and depression). Parents (often overprotective with no excess of marital discord) are aware and often collude. Treatment is graded or abrupt resumption of school attendance. Outcome is good in 60% of cases, although one-third have social difficulties and agoraphobia in adulthood.

20 Child Psychiatry II

Social functioning disorders

Elective (Selective) mutism (can be diagnosed at any age and is not included under most of 'child psychiatry', i.e. neurodevelopmental disorders)

• The child speaks fluently in familiar situations, such as home, but there is a lack of speech in less familiar settings, such as school, where there is an expectation of speaking.
• The disturbance interferes with educational or occupational achievement or with social communication.
• The duration is at least one month (not linked to the first month of school)
• The failure to speak is not attributable to lack of knowledge
• Affected children are usually very shy, withdrawn, with marked separation anxiety and a fear of social embarrassment. Two-thirds have language developmental delay.
• Prevalence is approximately 1/1000.
• Onset is typically in early childhood.
• Aetiology is genetic (increased family history of elective mutism and adult social phobia) and environmental (typically geographical or social isolation and anxious and overprotective parents).
• Long-term studies suggest that communication difficulties may extend into adulthood. The condition may be a precursor of adult social phobia.

Reactive attachment disorder

• This is characterised by persistent abnormalities in a child's pattern of relationships with parental figures and in other social situations; it usually develops before the age of 5. There are usually poor peer relations, fearfulness and hypervigilance that do not respond to reassurance, aggression towards self and others, misery, withdrawal and, in some cases, failure to thrive.
• Reactive attachment disorder arises from severe disturbance in the formation of early attachment relationships, often due to severe parental neglect, abuse or mishandling.
• Treatment seeks to achieve responsive, consistent parenting. This may require removing the child from the family.
• If unresolved, it may progress to conduct disorder or adult antisocial personality disorder.

Other disorders

Enuresis

• This is non-organic, involuntary bladder emptying after the age of 5 years. It can occur by day, by night or both, and is defined as secondary if there has been a period of urinary continence and primary if not.
• Prevalence is 10% at age 5, 5% at age 10 and 1% at age 18. It is twice as common in boys.
• Aetiological factors include positive family history, unsettling family events, developmental delay and other behavioural problems in the child.
• Management involves:
  • exclusion of physical pathology (especially urinary tract infection);

• addressing excessive or insufficient fluid intake or abnormal toileting patterns;
• reward systems (e.g. star charts) used to reinforce success, but the emphasis should be on adherence to the programme rather than to dryness;
• enuresis alarms: these devices are activated by moisture; alarms achieve dryness over time by training the child to recognise the need to pass urine and to wake to go to the toilet or hold on;
• medication: desmopressin (synthetic antidiuretic hormone) or imipramine (a tricyclic antidepressant) are sometimes prescribed.
• Ninety per cent of cases resolve by adolescence.

Encopresis

• The deposition of stool in inappropriate places in the presence of normal bowel control.
• Most children are faecally continent by 4 years. Prevalence of encopresis is about 2% in boys and 1% in girls at age 8 years.
• Encopresis may reflect anger (with deposits positioned to cause maximum distress to parents/carers) or regression in children unable to cope with the increasing independence expected of them. Voluntary faecal retention with subsequent overflow is present in some cases.
• Physical causes for constipation (e.g. Hirschsprung's disease) or pain on defecation must be ruled out.
• Encopresis is associated with emotional disturbance; intelligence is usually average or below average. There may be underlying parental marital conflicts, punitive potty training and/or sexual abuse.
• Treatment aims both to restore normal bowel habits and to improve parent/child relationships. Parents should be encouraged to ignore the soiling and in particular not to punish the child. More specific treatments include behaviour modification (e.g. star chart) and family therapy. Drug treatments are of very little use, except the use of laxatives if constipation is present.
• Ninety per cent of cases improve within one year and almost all resolve by adolescence. Associated conduct disorder may, however, persist.

Developmental/Neurodevelopmental disorders

Pervasive developmental disorders (PDD): is contained in ICD-10, but not DSM-5.

• These are among the most frequent childhood neurodevelopmental disorders, present in 60–70/10 000. They include:
  • autism
  • asperger's syndrome
  • childhood disintegrative disorder

Autistic Spectrum Disorder

• DSM-5 uses the term 'autism spectrum disorder' (ASD) to refer to all these disorders (ICD 10 lists them separately).

Psychiatry at a Glance, Sixth Edition. Cornelius Katona, Claudia Cooper, Mary Robertson. © 2016 John Wiley & Sons, Ltd. Published 2016 by John Wiley & Sons, Ltd.
Companion website: www.ataglanceseries.com/psychiatry

- This is present in about 20/10 000 children; it is more common in boys (3× more than in girls) and in social classes 1 and 2.
- The onset is before the age of 3 years and can even occur in the first few months. Three features are regarded as essential to the diagnosis:
  - a pervasive failure to make social relationships (aloofness, lack of eye contact, poor empathy, etc.), i.e. social–emotional reciprocity;
  - major difficulties/deficits with verbal and non-verbal communication/language development;
  - deficits in developing, maintaining, and understanding relationships;
  - resistance to change with associated ritualistic and/or manneristic behaviours.
- These may all reflect an inability to process emotional cues.
- Affected children often exhibit:
  - inappropriate attachments to unusual objects,
  - insistence on sameness,
  - a restricted range of interests and activities,
  - stereotyped behaviours (rocking, twirling, etc.),
  - hyper/hyporeactivity to sensory input,
  - unpredictable outbursts of screaming or laughter,
  - DSM-5 requires specification of severity.
- Ninety-five per cent have an IQ <95, but some have isolated skills (rote memory, computation).
- Learning disability, deafness and childhood schizophrenia must be considered in the differential diagnosis.
- Aetiological factors include:
  - genetic loading: associated genetic disorders include tuberous sclerosis and Fragile X syndrome;
  - perinatal complications.
- Treatment is with specialist, intensive (>25 hours a week) behavioural treatments. These typically:
  - break down skills (such as communication and cognitive skills) into small tasks, then teach those tasks in a highly structured way;
  - reward and reinforce positive behaviour;
  - discourage and redirect inappropriate behaviour.

Family support and counselling are crucial.
- Fifteen per cent achieve fully independent functioning as adults.
- Outcome is considerably better in those with a non-verbal IQ >70 and/or those in whom speech has developed by the age of 6 years.

Asperger's syndrome (included in ICD-10 not DSM-5)

- This is a less severe form of PDD with later onset, normal intelligence and language development and schizoid personality. Pedantic speech and a preoccupation with obscure facts often occur.

Childhood disintegrative disorder (disintegrative psychosis) (included in ICD 10, not included in DSM-5)

- This is very rare; prevalence is around 2/100 000.
- It is characterised by normal initial development (to age 4 years) and the subsequent onset of a dementia with social, language and motor regression with prominent stereotypes.
- The aetiology includes infections (especially subacute sclerosing panencephalitis) and neurometabolic disorders.

Specific developmental disorders

Specific reading (learning) retardation

- Reading difficulties that interfere with academic progress and are not accounted for by low intelligence, poor schooling or visual or auditory difficulties.

- Prevalence is between 5% and 10%, with a marked male and working-class preponderance.
- Neuropsychological testing often reveals perceptual and/or language deficits and there may be coexistent attention-deficit hyperactivity disorder (ADHD).
- Dyslexia is an alternative name

Psychotic disorders

- Psychoses of childhood are rare.
- Childhood schizophrenia may be acute in onset (carrying a better prognosis) or have a prodrome of apparent developmental delay.
- As in adolescence and adulthood, there is a genetic predisposition and the presentation is with hallucinations, delusions and thought disorder, but with a greater preponderance of motor disturbance, particularly catatonia.
- Antipsychotics are the mainstay of treatment, but the risk of weight gain and metabolic syndrome is particularly high in young people and vigilance to such side effects is crucial.
- Mania was thought not to occur before adolescence but is now increasingly recognised in the post-pubertal years.

Sleep problems

- These are common in normal children with night-time wakefulness in 20% and sleep-talking in 10%.
- DSM-5 refers to 'Sleep–wake disorders' including insomnia, hypersomnolence, narcolepsy, restless legs syndrome (not to be confused with akathisia), substance use disorders and those included below. In addition one must remember that sleep difficulties can be symptoms of ADHD (Chapter 19) and Tourette Syndrome (Chapter 29).
- Night terrors, in which children sit up terrified and screaming but cannot be woken sufficiently to be reassured, have a peak incidence (3%) at age 4–7 years and frequently a positive family history. They arise from deep (stage 4) sleep and are accompanied by tachycardia and tachypnoea. The incidences are aggravated by daytime stress and usually resolve spontaneously.
- Nightmares (peak incidence age 5–6 years) that occur during REM sleep may be equally frightening and are also often stress related, but the child can be easily woken and reassured.

Links between child and adult mental health

- There are strong links between childhood and adult mental health:

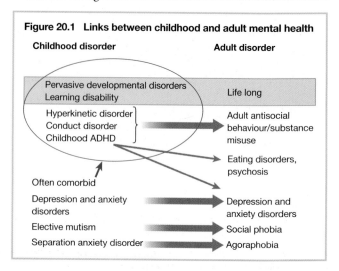

Figure 20.1 Links between childhood and adult mental health

21 The Psychiatry of Adolescence

Adolescence

• Adolescence starts with the onset of puberty and lasts until the attainment of full physical maturity.

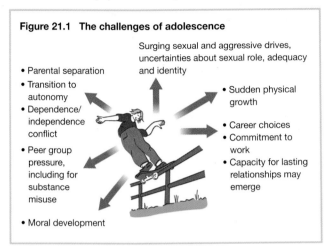

Figure 21.1 The challenges of adolescence

Surging sexual and aggressive drives, uncertainties about sexual role, adequacy and identity

• Parental separation
• Transition to autonomy
• Dependence/independence conflict
• Peer group pressure, including for substance misuse
• Moral development

• Sudden physical growth
• Career choices
• Commitment to work
• Capacity for lasting relationships may emerge

• About 13% of boys and 10% of girls aged 10–15 years have a psychiatric disorder.
• Conduct and hyperkinetic disorders ADHD are more common in boys and emotional disorders (mostly anxiety and depression) in girls.
• No psychiatric diagnoses are specific to adolescence; most adult and child psychiatric disorders are seen, often modified by the child's developmental stage.

Psychiatric assessment in adolescence

• Common presentations of psychiatric disorders in adolescence include emotional upset, identity issues, conflict with parents, delinquent behaviour and poor school performance.
• Comorbidity (between mental disorders and with substance misuse and self-harm) is even more common than in adults:

Figure 21.2 Mental disorders are often comorbid with each other, and with substance misuse and self-harm in adolescence

Mental disorders

Conduct disorders
Hyperkinetic disorders

Drug misuse
Alcohol misuse
Smoking

Depression
Anxiety disorders

Self-harm

Eating disorders

Note: Hyperkinetic = ICD-10;
DSM-5 = attention deficit hyperactivity disorder

• Level of functioning and apparent 'disorders' must be distinguished from developmental norms.

• Young people often do not acknowledge their own problems and parental and school involvement may cause conflict and distress. Trust and rapport must often be built up slowly in the face of resentment, suspicion and fear of being thought of as 'mad'.
• It is important to talk to the family to understand their perspective, as well as the family dynamics, which may be crucial in both aetiology and management.
• Developmental history is important because many adolescent disorders have clear childhood antecedents.
• The diagnostic process is the same as in adults, and DSM-IV-TR or ICD-10 classifications are used.

Conduct disorder

• Conduct disorder (see also Chapter 19) may emerge or worsen in adolescence.
• About one-third of adolescents with conduct disorder develop adult antisocial personality disorder.
• Psychosocial intervention should be the first line of treatment, along with treating comorbid disorders.
• If problems are severe, medication may be used cautiously.
  • Atypical antipsychotics (in particular risperidone, which is licensed for conduct disorder) may reduce aggressive behaviours, especially if there are coexisting neurodevelopmental disorders, such as autistic spectrum disorder.
  • Selective serotonin reuptake inhibitors (SSRIs) may reduce impulsivity, irritability and lability of mood.

Eating disorders (also see Chapter 13)

• Anorexia nervosa and bulimia nervosa are each found in about 1% of adolescents.
• Anorexia has its peak prevalence in adolescence and, if mild, may be difficult to distinguish from age-appropriate preoccupation with dieting.
• Adolescent-onset bulimia is increasingly common.

Mood disorders

• Mild episodes of depression (characterised by loneliness and low self-esteem) occur in 25% of adolescents, and moderate or severe depression in about 8%.
• Depression is about four times more common in adolescent girls.
• Clinical features are essentially the same as in adults, but poor appetite, weight loss and feelings of hopelessness may be more prominent than overt sadness; sleep is more often prolonged than disrupted.
• Interventions may include:
  • family therapy;
  • individual psychotherapy (particularly cognitive behavioural therapy; see Chapter 33);
  • antidepressants (see Chapter 35) may be indicated where biological features are prominent. Because of concerns that SSRIs may increase the risk of suicidal thoughts and self-harm, only fluoxetine is generally recommended for depression under the age of 18.

Psychiatry at a Glance, Sixth Edition. Cornelius Katona, Claudia Cooper, Mary Robertson. © 2016 John Wiley & Sons, Ltd. Published 2016 by John Wiley & Sons, Ltd.
Companion website: www.ataglanceseries.com/psychiatry

• Mania has a prevalence of up to 1% in adolescence; the presentation and management principles are similar to those for adults (see Chapter 9). Substance abuse and schizophrenia are the main differential diagnoses.

Anxiety, stress-related disorders

• Anxiety most frequently presents as overwhelming, non-specific worrying and repeated need and/or demand for reassurance.
• School refusal (as opposed to truancy) may arise from specific school-related phobias, anxiety or depression.
• Social phobias, characterised by avoiding contact with strangers, are also seen. Reassurance and advice (to adolescent, parents and school) on coping strategies and, in more serious cases, behavioural therapy, usually help (Chapter 33).
• Anxiety may also arise in response to stress; presentations and management of acute stress reaction and post-traumatic stress disorder (PTSD) are similar to adults.

Obsessive–compulsive disorder (OCD)

• Mild obsessionality is common in adolescence; true OCD may show prominent obsessional slowness and behaviour sufficiently bizarre to resemble schizophrenia. Resistance to the thoughts and behaviours may be absent.
• Treatment usually involves cognitive behavioural therapy.
• Where psychological treatment alone is not sufficient, SSRIs are recommended, with careful monitoring for side effects.
• OCD usually continues into adulthood (see also Chapter 12).

Schizophrenia

• The peak age of onset of schizophrenia is in late adolescence.
• Presentation is usually with deteriorating school performance; clinical features are otherwise as in adult life.
• In younger adolescents, initial presentation is often with:
  • bizarre behaviour
  • social withdrawal and anxiety
  • only fleeting first-rank symptoms.
• The differential diagnosis includes organic states, mood disorder, drug-induced psychosis, adolescent crises and schizoid personality.
• Atypical antipsychotics and rehabilitation are the mainstays of management. Given the limited safety data on antipsychotic use in youth, clinicians should be vigilant for side effects (see Chapter 34).

Self-harm

• Deliberate self-harm (DSH) is widespread in adolescents. It is more than twice as common among females as males. About 10% of girls aged 15–16 reported harming themselves in the previous year in a recent European survey. About half the young people decided to harm themselves in the hour before doing so, and many did not attend hospital or tell anyone else.
• It is often related to problems in relationships (family or friends) or problems with school or study.
• In the UK, over 90% of self-harm attempts involve overdoses, most often of paracetamol.
• Contagion (self-harming behaviour linked to peer-group influences) may be an important factor in DSH by adolescents, especially in girls who cut themselves.

• All children and young people who have harmed themselves should be admitted to a paediatric ward under the overall care of a paediatrician and assessed fully the following day.
• Actual suicide (particularly in boys and where there is coexistent substance abuse) has become more frequent in recent years, and the risk must be considered.

Substance abuse

• This is common in adolescence. Aetiology can include:
  • family and social adversity (or relative opulence)
  • vulnerable personality
  • peer pressure
  • associated conduct disorder or depression.
• The hallmarks of problematic abuse are:
  • abrupt deterioration in school performance (absenteeism, low grades, poor discipline);
  • lawbreaking, fights;
  • apparent personality change;
  • lethargy, lack of motivation, lack of concentration;
  • unexplained deterioration in physical health;
  • slurred speech, drowsiness.
• The patient usually denies any problems, and information from school or friends may therefore be vital.
• Depression and self-harm are frequent; the rise in adolescent suicide is largely accounted for by substance misuse.

Capacity and confidentiality

• The Mental Capacity Act (2005) in England and Wales and the Adults with Incapacity (Scotland) Act 2000 apply to people aged 16 and over. For those younger than 16, there is established case law governing consent to medical treatment.

Table 21.1 Who can give consent to medical treatment?

Under legal age of capacity*	On reaching legal age of capacity (adulthood)
Patient (young person) if a doctor judges they have the capacity to do so	**Patient only** If they lack capacity, capacity legislation applies as for all adults (Chapter 40)
Parent/legal guardian on child's behalf **The courts** can make child ward of court and overrule wishes of the parent and/or young person if they refuse to consent to treatment that doctors consider to be in the child's interests	

*aged 16 in England and Scotland; aged 18 in Northern Ireland

• The Mental Health Acts (see Chapters 40–42) may apply to a person of any age, but in practice children are usually treated informally with their consent or that of a parent.
• Health professionals are bound by duties of confidentiality to their patients and this includes young people.
• There are some exceptions to this, in particular if the patient or another person is at risk of harm (e.g. from an abuser).
• Respecting confidentiality does not mean that information should not be shared. Dialogue with parents and other carers and professionals is critical to care. It means professionals should seek consent to disclose information.

22 Learning Disability (Mental Retardation)

Figure 22.1   The two most common specific causes of LD

Down syndrome	Fragile X syndrome
1/700 live births (1/50 births to mothers aged 45+) Chromosome 21: 95% trisomy (▲ with maternal age) 5% translocation (can be inherited)	1/3600 males, 1/5000 females 8% of males with LD X-linked dominant condition Women have fewer learning and behavioural problems

Down syndrome

15% mild LD; other moderate or severe

5% autistic traits

Invariably Alzheimer's disease develops after age 50

▲ Hypothyroidism

50% have cardiac septal defects

Broad hands, single transverse palmar crease

Flat occiput

Oblique palpebral fissures

Small mouth

High arched palate

Fragile X syndrome

Most males and a third of affected females have LD

15–33% have autism

Large head and ears

Poor eye contact

Abnormal speech

Hypersensitivity to touch, auditory, visual stimuli

Hand flapping

Hand biting

Definition and epidemiology
- Learning disability (LD) comprises:
  - low intellectual performance,
  - onset at birth or in early childhood,
  - reduced life skills.
- About 1.5% of the population has an LD. This has not fallen despite recent reductions in the incidence of severe LD because of concurrent improvements in prevention (see below) and survival.

Aetiology
- Mild LD is not usually associated with specific causes and represents the lower end of the IQ normal distribution curve. IQ in general is strongly genetically determined, although the close correlation between parental and child IQ is also partly explained by shared social and educational deprivation.
- More severe LD is usually related to specific brain damage.
- Causes may be:
  - **genetic**:
    - chromosomal (e.g. Down, Klinefelter or Turner's syndrome);
    - X-linked: Fragile X, Lesch–Nyhan syndrome;
    - autosomal dominant: tuberose sclerosis, neurofibromatosis;
    - autosomal recessive: usually metabolic disorders (e.g. phenylketonuria).

Autism is usually associated with LD (Chapter 20).
- **antenatal**:
  - infective (e.g. toxoplasma, rubella and cytomegalovirus);
  - hypoxic, toxic or related to maternal disease.
- **perinatal**: prematurity, hypoxia, intracerebral bleed
- **postnatal**: infection, injury, malnutrition, hormonal, metabolic, toxic, epileptic.

Classification and clinical features
LD is classified as mild, moderate, severe and profound.

Psychiatric illness
- The prevalence of psychiatric disorders is increased in people with LD (although most people with LD do not have a psychiatric disorder). Reasons for this include the following factors:
  - genetic
  - organic (particularly epilepsy)
  - psychological (frustration)
  - social (such as stigma).
- Making specific psychiatric diagnoses can be difficult (particularly in people with moderate or severe LD) because of:
  - coexisting language deficits,
  - symptoms being attributed to the person's LD.
- **Psychological reactions** to adverse life events (such as bereavement) are often not recognised by carers.

Psychiatry at a Glance, Sixth Edition. Cornelius Katona, Claudia Cooper, Mary Robertson. © 2016 John Wiley & Sons, Ltd. Published 2016 by John Wiley & Sons, Ltd.
Companion website: www.ataglanceseries.com/psychiatry

Table 22.1 Severity and characteristics of LD

	Mild	Moderate	Severe	Profound
Defined as IQ of . . .	50–70	35–49	20–34	<20
Cause	Usually limited social/learning opportunities + genetic low IQ	Usually specific biological cause, e.g. Down syndrome, Fragile X syndrome		
Proportion of people with LD	80%	12%	7%	1%
Self care	Most live independently and can engage in some employment; difficulty coping with stress and more complex social functioning, e.g. parenting and handling money	Usually need supported accommodation or live with family	Very limited skills	
Language, motor and sensory abnormalities	Slight or absent 6% have epilepsy	Limited but useful language	Very limited language 33% have epilepsy 10% incontinent 15% cannot walk	

- Disorders with increased prevalence in LD include:
  - **behavioural disturbance**: more common with increasing severity of LD; occurs in <40% of children and 20% of adults with severe LD (e.g. purposeless or self-injurious behaviour, aggression or inappropriate sexual behaviour such as masturbation in public);
  - **depression**: diagnosis rests more on motor and behavioural changes (reduced sleep, retardation, tearfulness, etc.) than verbal expressions of distress;
  - **anxiety**: disorders (including obsessive–compulsive disorder and phobias);
  - **dissociative symptoms**: amnesia, episodes of unconsciousness, etc.;
  - **schizophrenia**: prevalence is 3% in LD and usually presents with simple and repetitive hallucinations and unelaborated, usually persecutory, delusions;
  - **mania**: usually presents as overactive/irritable behaviour.

Antenatal detection and prevention

- Antenatal genetic counselling and testing gives parents the option of termination of pregnancy (e.g. for Down syndrome).
- Improved perinatal care reduces the risk of brain injury.
- Early detection of hormonal or metabolic problems (myxoedema, phenylketonuria) may allow treatment before LD occurs.

Management

- Most people with LD now live in domestic homes, usually with their families.
- Support is provided by primary care, educational and social services. Specialist multidisciplinary community teams coordinate local services; assess and manage any concurrent mental illness, social skills and problem-solving training; and provide support with finances and accommodation.

- Children with mild LD usually receive educational support within mainstream schools; as adults, they may need support to access employment. Fewer people with LD than adults of normal intelligence with mental illness are in paid occupations.
- Treatment of mental illness is similar to that for patients without LD. Challenging behaviour is usually managed with behavioural therapy and changes to the individual's living situation and daily activities.
- People with LD need written information to be accessible (in a format they can understand). Those with more severe LD sometimes use Makaton, a communication system of signs and gestures.
- People with LD should be supported to make their own decisions if they can; if they cannot, decisions need to be made in their best interests, and capacity legislation applies (Chapter 40).
- It is important to be alert to potential reasons for psychological distress in people with LD. Common themes include:
  - realising that they may not achieve full independence,
  - realising that their parents are likely to die before they do,
  - issues around their sexuality.
- Sensitive, frank communication at a level the person with LD can understand is important.
- People with LD are at increased risk of physical, emotional and sexual abuse.

Communicating with people with learning disabilities

- Ask if they use a communication aid – they might have a communication passport that describes how they communicate.
- Listen carefully.
- Look at a person when he or she is talking.
- If you cannot understand, try to make the person feel at ease by saying, 'Sometimes it is difficult for me to understand. Could you say it again please?'
- Don't pretend to understand when you have not.
- Ask the person if it is okay to ask a carer/support worker for help with communication.

23 Cross-cultural Psychiatry

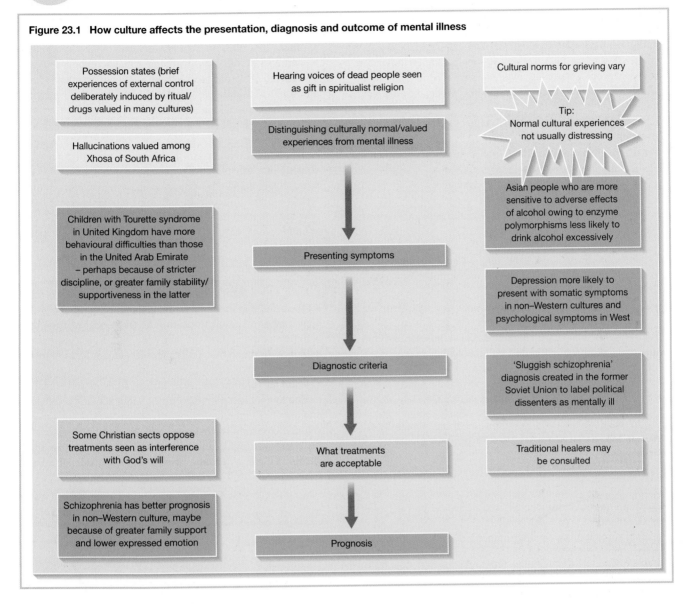

Figure 23.1 How culture affects the presentation, diagnosis and outcome of mental illness

Possession states (brief experiences of external control deliberately induced by ritual/drugs valued in many cultures)

Hallucinations valued among Xhosa of South Africa

Children with Tourette syndrome in United Kingdom have more behavioural difficulties than those in the United Arab Emirate – perhaps because of stricter discipline, or greater family stability/supportiveness in the latter

Some Christian sects oppose treatments seen as interference with God's will

Schizophrenia has better prognosis in non–Western culture, maybe because of greater family support and lower expressed emotion

Hearing voices of dead people seen as gift in spiritualist religion

Distinguishing culturally normal/valued experiences from mental illness

Presenting symptoms

Diagnostic criteria

What treatments are acceptable

Prognosis

Cultural norms for grieving vary

Tip: Normal cultural experiences not usually distressing

Asian people who are more sensitive to adverse effects of alcohol owing to enzyme polymorphisms less likely to drink alcohol excessively

Depression more likely to present with somatic symptoms in non–Western cultures and psychological symptoms in West

'Sluggish schizophrenia' diagnosis created in the former Soviet Union to label political dissenters as mentally ill

Traditional healers may be consulted

• Culture is the way that different groups of people perceive the world and interact with their environment. It incorporates patterns of social and family relationships and religious beliefs.

• Cross-cultural psychiatry examines concepts of mental health and illness and how symptomatology is culturally determined.

How culture can influence mental illness presentation and treatment

• Figure 23.1 shows how culture may affect the presentation, diagnosis and outcome of mental illness.

• It is important to consult someone knowledgeable in the relevant culture where there is doubt, to prevent misdiagnosing (or missing a diagnosis of) mental disorder.

Culture and standardised diagnosis

• The World Health Organization's International Pilot Study on Schizophrenia, carried out in the 1960s and 1970s, showed the following:

  • The prevalence of schizophrenia was remarkably stable across cultures.

  • Prognosis was better in non-Western societies. This may reflect greater availability of home support without high expressed emotion and the absence of a stigmatising label of chronic schizophrenia.

  • People with schizophrenia in Western developed countries showed a higher frequency of depressive symptoms, primary delusions, thought insertion and thought broadcasting, while in non-Western developing countries visual hallucinations were more frequent.

Psychiatry at a Glance, Sixth Edition. Cornelius Katona, Claudia Cooper, Mary Robertson. © 2016 John Wiley & Sons, Ltd. Published 2016 by John Wiley & Sons, Ltd.
Companion website: www.ataglanceseries.com/psychiatry

- Psychotic disorders (including psychotic depression and schizophrenia) were diagnosed reliably (using very similar criteria) in different cultures, but neurotic (anxiety/depression) and dissociative diagnoses were much less secure.

Mental illness and minority ethnic groups living in Western countries

- In the UK, the prevalence of schizophrenia is higher in African Caribbean people, especially those who are second generation, while the prevalence of schizophrenia in Caribbean countries is not raised.
- Irish people have particularly high rates of psychiatric hospital admissions.
- Putative explanations for these higher prevalences of mental illness in immigrant groups include:
  - higher rates of socioeconomic disadvantage;
  - racism;
  - the stress of migration (especially for refugees and asylum-seekers; see Chapter 24);
  - higher propensity for mental illness among those who move to another country;
  - misdiagnosis of affective disorders or cultural expressions of distress as schizophrenia;
  - differential responses by police, social and treatment services to some minority ethnic groups.
- South Asian women have a higher rate of overdoses than White British women. This might reflect 'culture conflict' in this group.
- Older African Caribbean people in the UK appear to be at greater risk of vascular dementia because of their higher prevalence of hypertension and other cardiovascular risk factors.

Racial differences in pharmacological response

Racial differences in distribution of enzyme polymorphisms explain:
- increased sensitivity to alcohol (and decreased prevalence of alcohol dependence) in Asian people;
- greater susceptibility to drug-induced dyskinesias in Asian people;
- higher plasma levels for given doses of tricyclic antidepressants and lithium in Black than White Americans, with resultant increased sensitivity to both therapeutic and adverse effects.

Culture-bound syndromes

- These denote patterns of symptoms or abnormal behaviour that are only recognised as illnesses in specific cultures.
- DSM-5 places the emphasis on 'cultural concepts of distress'. In ICD-10, they are coded according to the symptoms experienced (e.g. under dissociative or somatoform disorders; see Chapter 27).
- Many have been described, mostly representing somatic and/or dissociative responses to stress. They include the following.
  - **Amok**, described in Africa, Asia and New Guinea, is a response to humiliation involving initial brooding, followed by a period of altered consciousness with uncontrollable (usually homicidal and sometimes suicidal) rage, for which the subject has no subsequent memory. Traditionally, surviving sufferers were immune from legal redress, much as the French *crime passionnel*.
  - **Ataque de nervios** occurs in Hispanic American groups, and consists of a grief reaction characterised by fluctuating conscious level (often with subsequent amnesia), crying, shouting, trembling and difficulty in moving limbs. Hyperventilation may be important in precipitating symptoms.
  - **Latah**, which occurs in Asia and North Africa, is a response to intense stress characterised by altered consciousness, hypersuggestibility and mimicry (including echolalia and echopraxia).
  - **Koro**, found mainly in Asia, involves intense anxiety centred on the belief that the genitalia are retracting and that their disappearance will result in death. The traditional management is to tie a string around the penis and pull. Koro is associated with local tradition that ghosts have no genitals and is thus not delusional.
  - **Brain fag** is found mainly in African students and is characterised by concentration difficulties, vague somatic complaints and depressed mood.
  - Some 'Western' syndromes, including multiple personality disorder, overdosing, anorexia nervosa, bulimia nervosa and chronic fatigue syndrome, may also be considered culture bound.

Deaf culture

Some (but not all) people who are deaf or hard of hearing and use sign language identify themselves as culturally deaf. In deaf culture, sign language and the often close-knit social networks within the deaf community are valued, and deafness is not considered a condition that needs to be fixed. It is important that mental health professionals who treat deaf people have an awareness of the deaf community's subculture and their communication needs.

24 Psychiatry and Social Exclusion

• Socially excluded people face barriers accessing essential services or participating in everyday life. Exclusion usually results from multiple disadvantages and perhaps an inability to negotiate meeting complex needs arising from those disadvantages.

• People at risk of social exclusion include those who are homeless, prisoners, immigrants and people with disabilities or mental illness. Mental illness may be the cause or result of social exclusion.

• Those who are socially excluded can become trapped in a cycle of unemployment, poverty, crime, poor-quality accommodation or homelessness.

• In this chapter we look at the mental health of groups who are often socially excluded and discuss how mental health services have tried to reduce barriers to them accessing help for psychiatric disorders.

• In all these groups, people's socioeconomic status and experiences vary as much as in the general population. For example, asylum seekers are defined legally rather than on their plight, experience of asylum or status or income in their home country.

• The likelihood of experiencing a severe mental illness varies with gender (being more common in women) and degree of economic disadvantage in these groups as in the general population.

Homeless people (Figure 24.1)

• A minority of homeless people are rough sleepers; many more sleep in squats, night shelters, temporary accommodation or 'sofa-surf' on friends' floors.

• In many areas, dedicated teams provide psychiatric and medical care for homeless people, in hostels, day centres, outpatient centres and, where necessary, the street. This targeted, flexible outreach service can reach a far higher number of homeless people than conventional services and provide care that they find acceptable. It is, however, more expensive.

Refugees

• Nearly 1% of the world's population are refugees or displaced people. Asylum seekers are those waiting for the government to decide if they will be granted refugee status.

• Refugees have increased rates of anxiety, depression and post-traumatic stress disorder (PTSD) (<10% of refugees). High rates of suicide have been reported among asylum seekers held in detention or whose applications have been refused.

• Figure 24.2 shows the stresses that may increase the vulnerability of asylum seekers to mental illness. They may be held in detention centres; access to welfare and housing is restricted and they cannot legally work. Forced unemployment among asylum seekers can lead to disability from which they cannot recover because employment permits income and a positive role in a society where they may be seen as competitors for resources.

• Asylum seekers and refugees may face difficulties in accessing primary and (particularly) secondary health care, including psychiatric treatment because of language barriers or uncertainty over how to access help. Using interpreters where needed and providing information about how to access local services can help overcome these barriers.

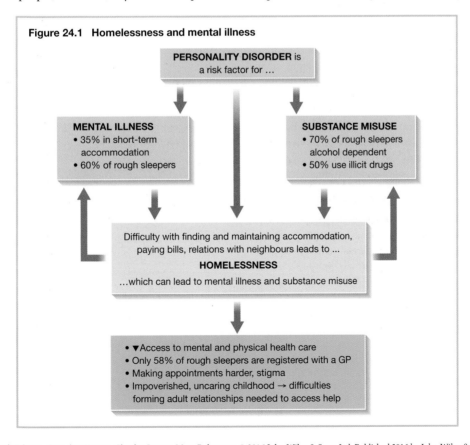

Figure 24.1 Homelessness and mental illness

PERSONALITY DISORDER is a risk factor for …

MENTAL ILLNESS
• 35% in short-term accommodation
• 60% of rough sleepers

SUBSTANCE MISUSE
• 70% of rough sleepers alcohol dependent
• 50% use illicit drugs

Difficulty with finding and maintaining accommodation, paying bills, relations with neighbours leads to …
HOMELESSNESS
…which can lead to mental illness and substance misuse

• ▼Access to mental and physical health care
• Only 58% of rough sleepers are registered with a GP
• Making appointments harder, stigma
• Impoverished, uncaring childhood → difficulties forming adult relationships needed to access help

Psychiatry at a Glance, Sixth Edition. Cornelius Katona, Claudia Cooper, Mary Robertson. © 2016 John Wiley & Sons, Ltd. Published 2016 by John Wiley & Sons, Ltd.
Companion website: www.ataglanceseries.com/psychiatry

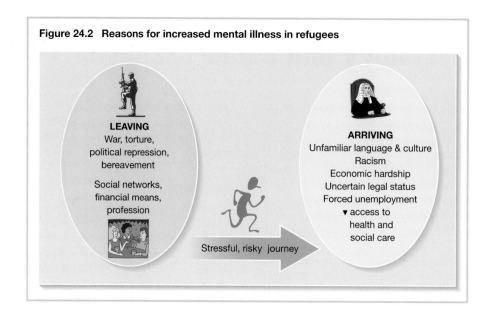

Figure 24.2 Reasons for increased mental illness in refugees

- Most applications for asylum in the UK are rejected, and those who remain after their application has been refused may be particularly vulnerable because they lose access to all benefits, accommodation, health and social care (except emergency care) and face deportation to the country from which they have fled.

Prisoners

- Figure 24.3 shows the high rates of mental illness in prison and the reasons for it. Despite serious attempts by the prison service to keep illicit substances out of prisons, over a third report using drugs during their prison term. Drug use is particularly high among people charged with burglary, robbery and theft, suggesting that the high costs of illicit drugs may be a factor in their criminality.
- People who have more social support, fewer recent stressful life events and who were working and married before entering prison are more likely to remain mentally healthy while in prison, but the proportion of such people in the prison system is low.
- In the past most psychiatric care in UK prisons was provided by prison doctors, who referred to local psychiatric services when required. In response to concerns that prisoners were receiving a lower standard of care than the general population, Community Mental Health In-Reach Teams have been set up in many prisons. People who have committed serious offences (murder, rape or serious violent offences) usually receive any psychiatric care required from regional forensic services.
- Prisoners who are seriously mentally ill cannot be compulsorily treated within the prison system in the UK, since the Mental Health Acts do not recognise prison hospital wings as hospitals.

These prisoners must be transferred to psychiatric (usually secure) units with agreement of the courts. High secure UK psychiatric facilities such as Broadmoor, Rampton and Ashworth are classified as hospitals, although they work in partnership with the prison system.

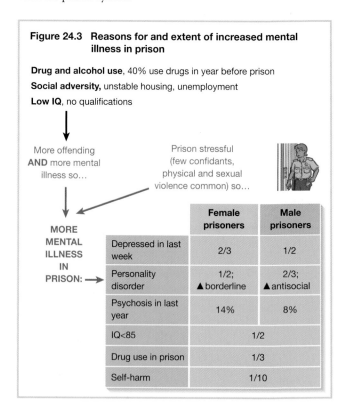

Figure 24.3 Reasons for and extent of increased mental illness in prison

Drug and alcohol use, 40% use drugs in year before prison

Social adversity, unstable housing, unemployment

Low IQ, no qualifications

More offending **AND** more mental illness so...

Prison stressful (few confidants, physical and sexual violence common) so...

MORE MENTAL ILLNESS IN PRISON:

	Female prisoners	Male prisoners
Depressed in last week	2/3	1/2
Personality disorder	1/2; ▲ borderline	2/3; ▲ antisocial
Psychosis in last year	14%	8%
IQ<85	1/2	
Drug use in prison	1/3	
Self-harm	1/10	

25 Psychiatry and Female Reproduction

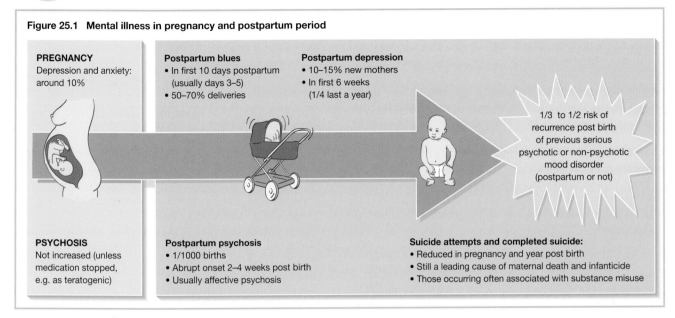

Figure 25.1 Mental illness in pregnancy and postpartum period

PREGNANCY
Depression and anxiety: around 10%

Postpartum blues
- In first 10 days postpartum (usually days 3–5)
- 50–70% deliveries

Postpartum depression
- 10–15% new mothers
- In first 6 weeks (1/4 last a year)

1/3 to 1/2 risk of recurrence post birth of previous serious psychotic or non-psychotic mood disorder (postpartum or not)

PSYCHOSIS
Not increased (unless medication stopped, e.g. as teratogenic)

Postpartum psychosis
- 1/1000 births
- Abrupt onset 2–4 weeks post birth
- Usually affective psychosis

Suicide attempts and completed suicide:
- Reduced in pregnancy and year post birth
- Still a leading cause of maternal death and infanticide
- Those occurring often associated with substance misuse

Mental illness during pregnancy

- Around 10% of pregnant women have significant depression or anxiety. It is more common in those with:
  - a past psychiatric history,
  - conflicting feelings about the pregnancy,
  - a history of sexual abuse as a child,
  - ultrasound scans showing fetal anomalies.
- The risk of psychosis is only increased if prophylactic medication is stopped, usually because of possible teratogenic effects.
- Alcohol and drug misuse often reduces in pregnancy.
- Alcohol, LSD and possibly cocaine are teratogenic.
- Opiates and alcohol can cause intrauterine growth retardation and withdrawal in the newborn.
- Suicide attempts may be reduced in pregnancy; those that occur are often associated with substance misuse.

Postpartum disorders

- Figure 25.1 shows the postpartum disorders, when they usually happen and how common they are.
- Risk of postpartum disorders appears similar after perinatal death (and less after abortion) to that after normal pregnancy and childbirth. Adequate opportunity to grieve should be provided, and bereavement counselling may be required. Formal psychiatric illness following termination of pregnancy is rare, but guilt feelings are common, need ventilating and may re-emerge in subsequent pregnancies.
- Women who have a history of serious mood disorder (affective disorder or affective psychosis), postpartum or otherwise, have a risk of recurrence after childbirth of between 1 in 2 and 1 in 3. Ask about psychiatric history prenatally to plan management.

Postpartum blues

- Postpartum blues are common and normal.
- The symptoms are emotional lability, crying, irritability and worries about coping with the baby.

- The cause is unclear; women with a history of premenstrual syndrome are at higher risk; elevated antepartum progesterone levels and precipitate postpartum falls in oestrogen, progesterone and sodium have been implicated.
- There is no clear relationship with obstetric or social variables.
- The blues are self-limiting, usually ending within a few days, but severe blues increase the risk of postpartum depression. No specific intervention is required (apart from reassurance), although, if symptoms do not resolve within two weeks, assess for depression.
- Appropriate antenatal education to warn expectant mothers and their partners about the blues is helpful.

Postpartum depression

- Clinical features are as for other depressive illness but may also include:
  - guilt and anxiety concerning the baby,
  - feelings of inadequate mothering,
  - unreasonable fears for the baby's health,
  - a reluctance to hold or feed the baby,
  - (more rarely) thoughts of harming the baby.
- It persists for a year or more in 25% of cases. Many cases are undetected.

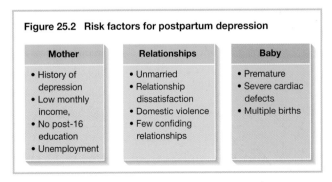

Figure 25.2 Risk factors for postpartum depression

Mother	Relationships	Baby
• History of depression • Low monthly income, • No post-16 education • Unemployment	• Unmarried • Relationship dissatisfaction • Domestic violence • Few confiding relationships	• Premature • Severe cardiac defects • Multiple births

Psychiatry at a Glance, Sixth Edition. Cornelius Katona, Claudia Cooper, Mary Robertson. © 2016 John Wiley & Sons, Ltd. Published 2016 by John Wiley & Sons, Ltd.
Companion website: www.ataglanceseries.com/psychiatry

Management involves full psychosocial assessment (including possible risk to mother and the baby).

• First line of treatment for mild to moderate perinatal depression is psychological therapy and not antidepressants because of the potential for adverse effects in the foetus or breastfeeding baby (see Table 25.1).

• Deliberate self-harm and suicide are less common in pregnancy and the postpartum year than at other times, but suicide is still one of the leading causes of maternal death in the UK and may be associated with infanticide.

• Interruption to the development of the mother–baby bond may occur; this is not specific to depression and may also occur in the context of ambivalence about the pregnancy or adverse life events. Prolonged maternal depression may also affect later social and cognitive development of the child, even after resolution of the maternal illness.

• About 10% of fathers also experience prenatal and postpartum depression. This is most common in the six months after the birth and is associated with maternal depression and relationship dissatisfaction.

Postpartum psychoses

• Risk appears highest:
  • in those with a previous episode of psychosis (postpartum or otherwise – see Figure 25.1),
  • in first-time mothers,
  • after instrumental delivery,
  • in those with a family history of affective disorder.
• Symptoms:
  • usually affective, most depressive but up to one-third manic (postpartum onset of schizophrenia is relatively unusual);
  • affective psychoses are often associated with Schneiderian first rank symptoms (Chapter 6);
  • emotional lability and subjective confusion are common.
• Assessment of suicide risk and of risk to the baby (who may suffer from neglect, inappropriate care, deliberate harm or even infanticide) is essential.

• Treatment usually requires hospitalisation, sometimes compulsorily, and, unless there are specific reasons not to do so, this should be with the baby to a specialist mother-and-baby unit.

• Treatment is usually with antipsychotics. Electroconvulsive therapy (ECT) has been reported to be particularly effective, irrespective of diagnostic group.

• Short-term prognosis is excellent.

Prescribing in pregnancy and during breastfeeding

• Antidepressants and antipsychotics are prescribed to many pregnant and breastfeeding women. We need to balance the risks of prescribing and not prescribing (Table 25.1).

• Breastfeeding women prescribed psychotropic drugs should be advised how to time feeds to avoid peak drug levels in milk and how to recognise adverse drug reactions in their babies.

• The evidence base is rapidly changing and specialist pharmacists or perinatal psychiatrists should be consulted where possible for updates on the current evidence.

• When prescribing **antidepressants**, consider that:
  • Tricyclic antidepressants, such as amitriptyline, imipramine and nortriptyline, have lower known risks during pregnancy than other antidepressants, but most tricyclic antidepressants have a higher fatal toxicity index than selective serotonin reuptake inhibitors (SSRIs).
  • Sertraline is the SSRI with the lowest known risk during pregnancy. Paroxetine should be avoided as it has been associated with fetal heart defects and neonatal pulmonary hypertension (as have other SSRIs to a lesser extent); SSRIs are associated with a neonatal behavioural syndrome.
  • All antidepressants carry the risk of withdrawal or toxicity in neonates; in most cases effects are mild.
  • Imipramine, nortriptyline and sertraline are present in breast milk at relatively low levels; citalopram and fluoxetine are present at relatively high levels.
• **Mood stabilisers** should be avoided where possible because:
  • Sodium valproate increases the risk of neural tube defects (from around 6 to 100–200 in 10 000) and can affect a child's intellectual development.
  • Carbamazepine increases the risk of neural tube defects (to around 20 to 50 in 10 000) and other major fetal malformations including gastrointestinal tract problems and cardiac abnormalities.
  • Lithium raises the risk of cardiac malformations from 0.8% to an estimated 6%.
  • They can have adverse effects in breast-fed infants.
• **Antipsychotics** are preferred to mood stabilisers for bipolar disorder. Low-dose typical antipsychotics such as haloperidol, chlorpromazine or trifluoperazine have the lowest known risks. Antipsychotics can induce an extrapyramidal syndrome in the baby. Olanzapine has been associated with gestational diabetes.
• **Benzodiazepines** can cause cleft palate and other fetal malformations, and 'floppy baby syndrome' in the neonate.

Premenstrual Dysphoric Disorder (PDD)

• Symptoms include low or labile mood, insomnia, poor concentration, irritability, poor impulse control, food craving and physical complaints (headache, breast tenderness and bloating).

• Onset is after ovulation, with improvement within a few days of the onset of menstrual flow.

• DSM-5 categorises it as PDD; ICD-10 lists it as a physical disorder.

• Up to 95% of women of reproductive age have some symptoms, but only 3–8% meet the criteria for PDD.

• Possible aetiological factors include a decrease in serotonin levels after ovulation, probably owing to interactions between oestrogen and serotonergic systems. Oestrogen may affect transcription of genes coding for synthesis of neurotransmitters and their receptors.

Table 25.1 The risks of prescribing and not prescribing

	In pregnancy	In postnatal period
Risks of prescribing	Teratogenic effects, withdrawal or toxicity in neonates	Adverse drug reactions in breastfeeding infants
Risks of not prescribing	Impact on foetus and mother of: disturbed behavior; stress; suicidal behaviour	Depression can affect: maternal–child bonding; child development

26 Functional Psychiatric Disorders in Old Age

- Older people may suffer from the same functional psychiatric disorders as younger adults (mood, anxiety and psychotic disorders), and the presentation and management of these are essentially the same as earlier in life.
- Older people continue to manifest personality disorders.
  - The degree of distress and disability caused by impulsive and antisocial traits often decreases with age.
  - Other traits may cause particular difficulty in negotiating the challenges of old age (e.g. people with schizoid traits may be less willing to accept home care, and people with anxious traits may have particular difficulty coping with chronic illness).

Depression in old age
Epidemiology and clinical features

- Increased age is not linked with higher rates of depression, which affects around 13% of older people. Depression is more common in those with physical illnesses and/or dementia.
- Older people with depression are less likely to receive treatment with antidepressants or talking therapy, even though they frequently consult their GP. This is partly because of the unjustified idea that depression is an inevitable consequence of ageing and also because of important differences in clinical presentation.
- Older people with depression are less likely than younger people to report low mood; they may present needing help but with presenting complaints other than low mood.
- They are also less likely to express suicidal ideation despite being at substantially higher risk of completed suicide.
- Compared with younger adults, depression in older adults is more likely to present with:
  - disturbed sleep (but decreased sleep duration occurs in normal ageing);
  - multiple physical problems for which no cause can be found;
  - motor disturbance (retardation and/or agitation);
  - dependency having previously been independent.

Aetiology

- Genetic factors are significant, although family history is less often positive than in younger depressed patients.
- People who become depressed for the first time in late life are more likely to have brain-imaging abnormalities and poor treatment response. This suggests that late first-onset depression may, in some cases, reflect the onset of neurodegenerative changes.
- Dementia is a risk factor for developing depression.
- There is a well-documented association between vascular risk factors and depression in later life; about 20% of people with coronary artery disease develop depression.
- Loss(es), such as bereavement, deteriorating physical health or financial insecurity may lead to depression. A third of older people live alone; many are socially isolated and lack confiding relationships.
- Being in residential or nursing care doubles the risk of depression in old age.
- Depression is increased in carers of people with dementia.

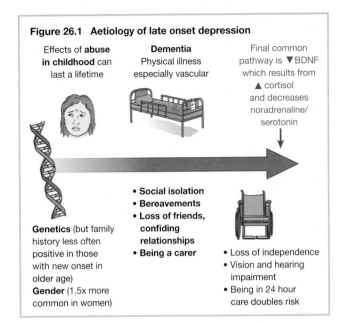

Figure 26.1 Aetiology of late onset depression

Effects of **abuse in childhood** can last a lifetime

Dementia Physical illness especially vascular

Final common pathway is ▼BDNF which results from ▲cortisol and decreases noradrenaline/ serotonin

Genetics (but family history less often positive in those with new onset in older age)
Gender (1.5x more common in women)

- Social isolation
- Bereavements
- Loss of friends, confiding relationships
- Being a carer

- Loss of independence
- Vision and hearing impairment
- Being in 24 hour care doubles risk

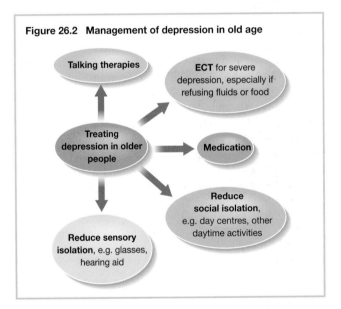

Figure 26.2 Management of depression in old age

Talking therapies

ECT for severe depression, especially if refusing fluids or food

Treating depression in older people

Medication

Reduce social isolation, e.g. day centres, other daytime activities

Reduce sensory isolation, e.g. glasses, hearing aid

Management

- Both physical and psychological treatments are effective, but they are underused in older people.
- Reducing social and sensory isolation may be important (through, for example, hearing aids and glasses, and day centre referral).
- Cognitive behavioural therapy may need to be modified to the needs of an older group but is effective in group as well as individual settings. In dementia, the focus may be on behavioural management and working with carers.
- Antidepressants with a relative lack of contraindications and favourable side-effect profiles, including selective serotonin reuptake inhibitors (SSRIs), venlafaxine and mirtazapine, have

been critical for the effective treatment of depression in older people, though randomised placebo-controlled trial evidence for efficacy is limited.

• Tricyclic antidepressants are effective but usually avoided because of the higher risk of clinically important side effects, particularly postural hypotension and resultant falls.

• Lithium augmentation is effective in some older patients with refractory depression.

• Adherence to antidepressant treatment may be difficult to achieve in older people, particularly since they may take longer (up to eight weeks) to take effect. However, if there is little or no response to an adequate antidepressant at four weeks, a switch to an antidepressant from a different class should be considered.

• There is new evidence that antidepressants are not effective in dementia (so consider other treatment first unless severe depression/risk of suicide).

• Electroconvulsive therapy (ECT) is very effective in more severe depression, particularly in patients with delusions or psychomotor retardation and those refusing food or fluid, in whom the risk of irreversible physical deterioration is high.

Prognosis

• Depression doubles the mortality rate in older people. Factors explaining this include:
  • medical morbidity – related to hypercortisolaemia in chronic depression, decreased exercise, non-adherence to medication, and self-neglect;
  • increased risk of suicide, especially in older depressed men.

• The prognosis is improved by early intervention, because longer duration of depressive episode predicts poor outcome. There is a high risk of chronicity (about 50% if untreated) and of relapse. Secondary prevention (continuing antidepressant therapy to prevent relapse) is highly effective.

Anxiety disorders

• General anxiety is often coexistent with (and responsive to the same treatment approaches as) depression.

• New episodes of phobic disorder, particularly agoraphobia, are often precipitated by traumatic events (e.g. a fall).

Mania in old age

• Mania accounts for about 20% of all psychiatric admissions for affective disorders in older people. Most have a past history of depression.

• In about 20% of cases, new onset mania in older age is precipitated by acute physical illness such as stroke.

• A tenth of new onset cases of mania occur over the age of 60.

• Overt elation is less often present than in mania in earlier life, although the patient generally has grandiose ideation. The clinical picture more usually consists of irritability, lability of mood and perplexity, much like that of delirium (see Chapter 31) but distinguishable by clear consciousness.

• Antipsychotics are effective in acute treatment, and some (e.g. olanzapine) are affective at preventing relapse, but atypical antipsychotics must be used with particular caution in people with dementia or vascular risk factors because of increased risks of stroke (see Chapter 34).

• Lithium may be used both acutely and in prophylaxis, although as many as 25% of older people (particularly those with Parkinson's disease or dementia) develop neurotoxicity. Both therapeutic and toxic effects of lithium may occur at lower blood levels in old age, so close monitoring is needed.

• The prognosis with treatment is good, although recurrence occurs in up to 50% by ten years.

Psychotic disorders

• Older people with psychosis may have illnesses that have continued from earlier in life or be presenting with a first episode.

• Symptoms are as for younger adults.

• There is a second peak in the incidence of schizophrenia over the age of 60.

• ICD-10 and DSM-5 do not distinguish between illnesses with onset in early and later life, but according to consensus:
  • *late onset schizophrenia* = onset age 40 to 60;
  • *very late onset schizophrenia* = onset age 60+.

• Aetiological factors include:
  • a genetic component (with excess family history of psychiatric illness and particularly schizophrenia);
  • sensory deprivation (particularly deafness);
  • social isolation – people who have had few relationships often become isolated with retirement or immobility or occasionally loss of a partner in older age;
  • brain imaging abnormalities in schizophrenia as in younger people;
  • organic brain disease and underlying physical illness.

Figure 26.3 describes the aetiology of late onset psychosis.

• Treatment is often difficult because of lack of insight, but response to antipsychotics, combined if possible with social reintegration, is usually good. As older people are at particular risk of tardive dyskinesia, atypical antipsychotics are recommended.

• Relapse is frequent if antipsychotics are withdrawn.

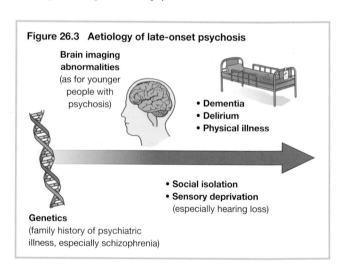

Figure 26.3 Aetiology of late-onset psychosis

Brain imaging abnormalities (as for younger people with psychosis)

• **Dementia**
• **Delirium**
• **Physical illness**

• **Social isolation**
• **Sensory deprivation** (especially hearing loss)

Genetics (family history of psychiatric illness, especially schizophrenia)

The Interface of Psychiatry and Physical Illness

Part 5

Chapters

27 Psychiatry and Physical Illness

Comorbidity of psychiatric and physical illness

• Psychiatric morbidity (consisting mainly of dementia, delirium, depression and anxiety) is present in 25–45% of inpatients, irrespective of their primary diagnosis. Figure 27.1 shows the reasons for this high comorbidity.

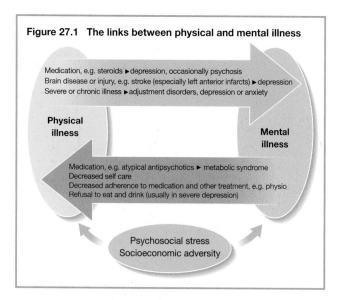

Figure 27.1 The links between physical and mental illness

Medication, e.g. steroids ▶ depression, occasionally psychosis
Brain disease or injury, e.g. stroke (especially left anterior infarcts) ▶ depression
Severe or chronic illness ▶ adjustment disorders, depression or anxiety

Physical illness → **Mental illness**

Medication, e.g. atypical antipsychotics ▶ metabolic syndrome
Decreased self care
Decreased adherence to medication and other treatment, e.g. physio
Refusal to eat and drink (usually in severe depression)

Psychosocial stress
Socioeconomic adversity

Some personality traits may worsen outcomes from illnesses; for example, individuals with 'Type D personalities' (pessimism, worry, social inhibition) do worse following myocardial infarction.

• Psychological therapies such as cognitive behavioural therapy (CBT) may help people live with illness and its treatment.

• As many as 30% of acute medical patients have some cognitive deficits, reflecting in part the vulnerability of older people to both cognitive and physical disorders.

• Dementia (see Chapter 32) may first become apparent during hospitalisation as patients reveal their inability to learn to cope in a novel environment and without family support. Dementia is associated with increased length of hospital stay, and early detection helps in planning discharge.

• Some symptoms of serious physical illness (such as lethargy, poor sleep and reduced appetite) can be difficult to distinguish from those of depression. It can help to focus on emotional features such as anhedonia, guilt and hopelessness. Antidepressants may be beneficial. Electroconvulsive therapy (ECT) can be life-saving in severe or psychotic depressive illness in physically ill people, particularly where suicidal risk is high or where physical health is further threatened by poor food and fluid intake.

• Patients with **pre-existing psychiatric illness** may require urgent medical or surgical management. Such patients will need continued psychiatric management with careful monitoring of their mental state under stressful circumstances.

Liaison psychiatry

• The overlap of psychiatric and physical symptoms requires close cooperation between psychiatric and medical staff. In medical and surgical wards and clinics, this is managed through the liaison psychiatry team.

• Patients presenting with behavioural disturbance frequently have delirium (which must be excluded, or its underlying cause identified and treated as a matter of urgency) or dementia.

• Suicidal threats or acts may cause medical/surgical staff considerable anxiety; they may need advice on assessing and managing suicide risk (Chapter 5).

• Multidisciplinary discussion of behavioural problems can identify triggers to undesirable behaviour and help find ways of defusing provocative situations.

Medically unexplained symptoms

Many people experience medical symptoms for which no cause is found. Here are the possible explanations.

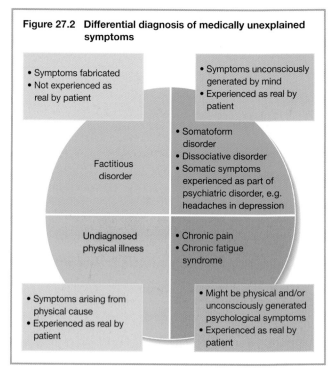

Figure 27.2 Differential diagnosis of medically unexplained symptoms

• Symptoms fabricated
• Not experienced as real by patient

• Symptoms unconsciously generated by mind
• Experienced as real by patient

Factitious disorder

• Somatoform disorder
• Dissociative disorder
• Somatic symptoms experienced as part of psychiatric disorder, e.g. headaches in depression

Undiagnosed physical illness

• Chronic pain
• Chronic fatigue syndrome

• Symptoms arising from physical cause
• Experienced as real by patient

• Might be physical and/or unconsciously generated psychological symptoms
• Experienced as real by patient

• When treating medically unexplained symptoms, be as honest and open as possible with the patient, acknowledge the symptoms and try not to let frustration or anger affect your management. Communication with the GP and other professionals involved in the patient's care can prevent the replication of investigations and ensure consistency.

Psychiatry at a Glance, Sixth Edition. Cornelius Katona, Claudia Cooper, Mary Robertson. © 2016 John Wiley & Sons, Ltd. Published 2016 by John Wiley & Sons, Ltd.
Companion website: www.ataglanceseries.com/psychiatry

Somatoform disorders

A quarter of GP attendees have somatoform disorders. These include somatisation disorder and hypochondriacal disorder.

Somatisation disorder

• This is characterised in ICD-10 by at least two years of multiple physical symptoms with no physical explanation; patients persistently refuse to accept the advice of doctors that there is no physical explanation, and their social and family functioning is impaired as a result of the illness.
• Gastrointestinal and skin complaints are the most common.
• Somatisation disorder is much more common in women than in men, usually starting before the age of 30.

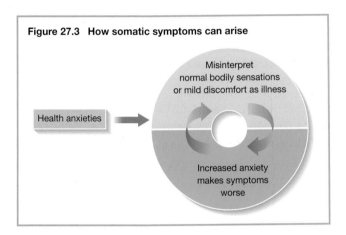

Figure 27.3 How somatic symptoms can arise

• It sometimes results in multiple operations despite the absence of organic disorder.
• Figure 27.3 explains how symptoms may arise. Patients are not consciously aware of the origin of their symptoms, no matter how clear and sometimes frustrating this might be to their families and carers.
• Treatment should begin by ruling out all organic illnesses.

Hypochondriacal disorder

• This is a non-delusional preoccupation with the possibility of serious illness such as cancer, heart disease, HIV or AIDS, despite medical reassurance.
• It is more common in men and people who have more contact with disease (e.g. health workers).
• **Dysmorphophobia** is related to hypochondriacal disorder. It is an excessive preoccupation with imagined or barely noticeable defects in physical appearance. For example, patients may become preoccupied by the size of their nose, believing an objectively normal nose to be ugly and deformed. This may lead to avoidance behaviour.

Many think it is on a spectrum with obsessive–compulsive disorder.
• Cognitive behavioural therapy (CBT) is the mainstay of treatment for somatoform disorders together with a focus on psychosocial and not physical symptoms. SSRIs can be helpful for dysmorphophobia.

Dissociative disorders (also termed 'conversion disorders')

• In dissociative disorders, physical (almost always neurological) symptoms occur in the absence of pathology and have a clear relationship with stressful events or disturbed relationships. Diagnoses include:

dissociative motor and sensory deficits	e.g. limb weakness, numbness, blindness
dissociative convulsions (non-epileptic seizures)	present in 9–50% of patients referred to specialist epilepsy centres; they can co-occur with epileptic seizures
dissociative amnesia	usually upsetting and personal information is forgotten
dissociative fugue	where dissociative amnesia is associated with a seemingly purposeful unplanned journey away from home
Ganser's syndrome	see Chapter 16

• The traditional psychoanalytic view suggests that in dissociative (conversion) disorders painful memories or thoughts (or the distress associated with them) are 'cut off' from the conscious self (Freud used the term 'repressed memories') and 'converted' into more acceptable and bearable physical symptoms. This is called 'primary gain'. Other psychological views see conversion disorders as resulting from ineffective communication.
• Although rare in the general population, dissociative disorders affect between 4% and 30% of neurology outpatients; they are more common in women.
• Management involves ensuring that there really is no organic basis, treating any underlying mood disorder and exploring with the patient and the family any 'secondary gain' (such as sympathy or avoidance of family conflict) that might be maintaining symptoms.
• Dissociative disorders differ from somatisation in that they more often present with signs rather than only symptoms and are often acute in their presentation.
• Thinking about the distinction between dissociative and hypochondriacal and somatisation disorders can be confusing; here are some tips about how to tell them apart.

Table 27.1 Distinguishing somatisation disorder, hypochondriacal and dissociative disorders

	Somatisation disorder	Hypochondriacal disorder	Dissociative disorder
Most commonly presents with	Physical symptoms – most often gastrointestinal or skin complaints	Fear of having a serious illness, e.g. cancer or AIDS	Neurological signs, e.g. paralysis, amnesia
Wants	A diagnosis to explain symptoms	The all clear (or worst fears confirmed so can have treatment)	A diagnosis to explain signs
Might say	*I've got all these pains. Why can't the doctor find out what is wrong with me?*	*I know I've got cancer; they just haven't done the right test yet.*	*What is happening to me?*

Table 27.2 DSM 5 categorisation of the disorders in this chapter

Dissociative Disorders	Dissociative Identity Disorder
	Dissociative Amnesia
	Depersonalisation/ Derealisation Disorder
	Specified & Unspecified Dissociative Disorders
Somatic Symptom & Related Disorders	Somatic Symptom Disorder
	Illness Anxiety Disorder
	Conversion Disorder (8 subtypes) (Functional Neurological Symptom Disorder)
	Psychological factors affecting other medical conditions
	Factitious Disorder - on self or by proxy
	Other specified & unspecified Symptom and Related Disorders

Factitious disorder

• In contrast to somatoform and dissociative disorders, people with factitious disorder deliberately feign or actually induce illness in themselves. Munchausen's syndrome is another name for it.
• The patient's reasons for feigning an illness are often complicated and may relate to
  • the gaining of nurture from others,
  • tangible benefit (e.g. avoiding criminal sanction, work or school).

Managing pain and fatigue

• Pain may trigger psychiatric referral even without clear evidence of somatoform disorder.
• Depression may underlie such pain or result from it, particularly if pain is inadequately treated for fear of causing opiate dependence. Chronic pain may respond to psychological therapy and antidepressants even in the absence of clear-cut depression.
• Chronic fatigue syndrome (also called ME or myalgic encephalomyelitis) is characterised by exhaustion after minimal physical activity, poor concentration and muscle tenderness. Recommended first-line treatment is CBT and/or graded exercise therapy.

DSM 5 categorises the disorders in this chapter somewhat differently, as shown in Table 27.2

28 Neuropsychiatry I

• Neuropsychiatry concerns conditions in which mental disorder results from demonstrable structural or neurophysiological disturbance of the brain. Another definition is 'the disorders which straddle the boundaries between neurology and psychiatry' (e.g. Tourette's Syndrome, Parkinson's Disease, Huntington's Disease, epilepsy).

• The psychiatric picture seldom bears a specific relationship to the type of underlying pathology, being more influenced by the site of brain involvement and the time course of the illness. It may include:
  • personality and behavioural changes
  • cognitive impairment and confusional states
  • affective disturbances
  • psychoses.

• An organic disorder can mimic functional disorders. The features below suggest organic problems.

Fluctuating symptoms
Localised (specific) cognitive deficits
Associated neurological signs
Vague or transient paranoid delusions
Olfactory or visual hallucinations

Untypical symptoms of a functional disorder
Record of cognitive disorder before other psychiatric symptoms

• A history, mental state examination and full physical and neurological exams are all needed to make the diagnosis.

• Investigations should include a general screen (see Chapter 31).

• More specialised investigations may help to confirm or exclude specific diagnoses.

• Lumbar puncture should be undertaken with caution if raised intracranial pressure is suspected, in view of the risk of precipitating brainstem coning.

Focal neurological disorders: traumatic brain injuries and strokes

• The neuropsychiatric presentations of cerebrovascular accidents (CVA; strokes) and traumatic brain injuries (TBI) are similar so they are considered together. In both conditions, acute focal brain injuries result in neurological disability followed by a recovery period.

• Acute effects include disturbance of consciousness, amnesia and behavioural disorder. Worse cognitive outcomes are associated with:
  • longer duration of post-traumatic amnesia (loss of memories about the injury and subsequent events), this is a more accurate prognostic indicator than retrograde amnesia (loss of memories from before the injury);
  • duration of loss of consciousness greater than 24 hours.

• Figure 28.1 describes the psychiatric sequelae of CVAs and TBIs. The aetiology of these involves:
  • direct neurophysiological effects (e.g. the cognitive disorders, temporal lobe injuries and psychosis);

• the psychosocial impact of sudden disability (important in anxiety and depression, although these may also relate directly to the injury).

• Lability of mood and apathy may be particularly prominent.

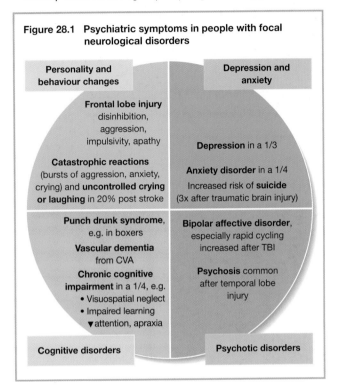

Figure 28.1 Psychiatric symptoms in people with focal neurological disorders

Personality and behaviour changes

Frontal lobe injury disinhibition, aggression, impulsivity, apathy

Catastrophic reactions (bursts of aggression, anxiety, crying) and **uncontrolled crying or laughing** in 20% post stroke

Depression and anxiety

Depression in a 1/3

Anxiety disorder in a 1/4

Increased risk of **suicide** (3x after traumatic brain injury)

Punch drunk syndrome, e.g. in boxers

Vascular dementia from CVA

Chronic cognitive impairment in a 1/4, e.g.
• Visuospatial neglect
• Impaired learning
▼attention, apraxia

Bipolar affective disorder, especially rapid cycling increased after TBI

Psychosis common after temporal lobe injury

Cognitive disorders

Psychotic disorders

Post-concussional syndrome

• A 'post-concussional syndrome' has been described after head injury, characterised by:

Anxiety	Depression
Irritability	Emotional lability
Insomnia	Hypersensitivity to noise/light
Reduced concentration	Chronic tiredness

• There may be an organic basis for the syndrome, but psychological and social factors are likely to play a major role.

• There is no specific treatment.

Epilepsy

• The prevalence of epilepsy is 0.5–1%, excluding febrile convulsions, single seizures and inactive cases.

• It is slightly more common in men.

• In most cases the cause is unknown.

• Known causes include:
  • cerebrovascular disease (15%)
  • cerebral tumours (6%)
  • alcohol-related seizures (6%)
  • post-traumatic seizures (2%).

Psychiatry at a Glance, Sixth Edition. Cornelius Katona, Claudia Cooper, Mary Robertson. © 2016 John Wiley & Sons, Ltd. Published 2016 by John Wiley & Sons, Ltd.
Companion website: www.ataglanceseries.com/psychiatry

- Onset is usually before the age of 30 (75%); however, the prevalence is increasing as the population ages because the prevalence of cerebrovascular disease is higher in older people.
- The most common seizure type is complex focal (60%), 60% of which arise in the temporal lobes.
- Epilepsy is present in around 25% of people with intellectual disability.
- Psychiatric aspects of epilepsy may be divided into:
  - preictal (before the seizure)
  - ictal (during)
  - postictal (afterwards)
  - interictal (disturbances are chronic and not related to the ictal electric discharge).
- Figure 28.2 shows when depression and psychosis usually occur in relation to seizures.

Figure 28.2 Relationship of depression and psychosis to seizures

	Depression	Psychosis
Pre-ictal	Can occur	Rare
Ictal	Can occur	Rarely occurs as part of simple partial, complex partial, or absence seizures
Post-ictal	Relatively common	• In 6–10% with intractable epilepsy: begins <1 week post seizure • Lasts hours → months
Inter-ictal	Very common	• Can develop in those with recurrent post-ictal episodes; usually associated with TLE • Symptoms very similar to schizophrenia

Depression

- Depression affects 30–50% of people with epilepsy at some time.
- Aetiological factors include:
  - demoralisation, stigma;
  - possibly lesion location (e.g. higher rates in temporal lobe epilepsy (TLE);
  - anti-epileptic drugs (e.g. phenobarbitone and vigabatrin);
  - a family history of depression;
  - adverse life events, financial stress and unemployment.
- Depression can directly increase seizure frequency through the mechanism of sleep deprivation.
- Treatment includes careful use of antidepressants.
  - Selective noradrenaline and serotonin reuptake inhibitors (SNRIs) and selective serotonin reuptake inhibitors (SSRIs) are recommended as least likely to lower the seizure threshold.
  - Citalopram is also least likely to interact with anti-epilepsy drugs.
- Electroconvulsive therapy (ECT) may be given if necessary.
- Carbamazepine and lamotrigine are anti-epileptic agents that may also improve mood.
- Suicide is five times higher in people with epilepsy and 25 times higher in people with temporal lobe epilepsy compared with the general population.

Panic disorder

- Panic disorder has a lifetime prevalence of 21%. It can be inter-ictal or peri-ictal; it is important not to mistake seizure activity for panic.

Psychosis

- Psychosis occurs in 3–7% of people with epilepsy.
- It is most commonly postictal.
- Postictal psychosis should be distinguished from delirium. It occurs up to a week after the seizure and lasts from as little as a day up to three months. Symptoms may include delusions, depressive or manic psychosis, or bizarre thoughts and behaviour. Visual hallucinations are common.
- Psychosis is more common with partial epilepsies and temporal lobe damage.
- Treatment is with antipsychotics, preferably those with least effect on seizure threshold (e.g. sulpiride, haloperidol).

Cognitive impairments

- Cognitive impairments are common in people with epilepsy and may be caused by:
  - anti-epileptic medication (phenobarbitone, phenytoin),
  - persistent abnormal electrical activity in the brain between seizures.

Sexual dysfunction

- Sexual dysfunction is common in people with epilepsy; causes include:
  - anti-epileptic medication side effects,
  - neurophysiological problems (more common in TLE),
  - social problems.

Pseudoseizures

- Also called dissociative convulsions (Chapter 27).
- They simulate real seizures and occur in 20–30% of people with chronic treatment-resistant epilepsy.
- They often:
  - occur frequently;
  - occur when other people are present, indoors or at home;
  - have an emotional precipitant;
  - are associated with a history of childhood sexual abuse.
- Characteristically, the electroencephalogram (EEG) is normal during the attack.

Tumour

- Primary and secondary intracranial tumours can lead to behavioural, affective, psychotic, personality and cognitive disturbances via a number of mechanisms, including mass effects and obstructive hydrocephalus.
- Malignancy outside the cranium can also lead to neuropsychiatric disturbance as a result of tumour by-products or effects on renal, endocrine and other body systems.

Note: In ICD-10 depressive disorders due to another medical condition are coded under the specific physical disorder. DSM-5 has a code for Depressive Disorder Due to Another Medical Condition (293.83), and the name of the other medical condition is noted.

29 Neuropsychiatry II

Autoimmune and inflammatory disorders

Multiple sclerosis

• Multiple sclerosis (MS) is the most common cause of neurological disability in working-age adults. Episodes of demyelination result in central nervous system abnormalities.
• Aetiology is unknown, with genetic and environmental factors (e.g. virus) probably important.
• The table shows the psychiatric complications of MS.

Table 29.1 Psychiatric complications of multiple sclerosis and their likely cause

Psychiatric complication	Likely cause
Cognitive deficits, dementia	Disease process (demyelination)
Depression	Stress rather than disease process; steroids, baclofen, beta interferon
Mania	Disease process
	Drugs (steroids, baclofen)
Euphoria/elation, emotional lability, pathological laughing/crying (10%)	Disease process

• The suicide rate is doubled in MS compared with the general population; rates are higher in people with alcohol problems and depression and in those who live alone.
• The prevalences of depression (25–50% in lifetime) and bipolar affective disorder are increased, but non-affective psychosis is no more common. People with psychosis (affective or non-affective) and MS are more likely to have plaques in bilateral temporal horn areas.
• Emotional lability (20%), elation/euphoria (elevated mood without overactivity – in 25%) and pathological laughing or crying (exaggerated emotional responses without associated feelings of distress – in 10%) all occur.
• Cognitive deficits are present in up to half of people with MS.
  • They arise early in the illness and usually progress slowly, although risk factors for a more rapid decline include more rapid disease progression and older age.
  • Particular impairment is seen in:
    – verbal fluency
    – comprehension
    – naming
    – executive functioning
    – memory.
  • They are usually associated with emotional lability and decreased information-processing speed.
• Subcortical dementia also occurs, usually late in the illness.

Systemic lupus erythematosus

• Systemic lupus erythematosus (SLE) is an autoimmune disorder that often affects the brain and nervous system (>50%).
• The table shows the psychiatric complications and their likely causes.

Table 29.2 Psychiatric complications of SLE and their likely cause

	Cause
Cognitive impairments	Disease process, usually acute confusional states (e.g. due to CNS vasculitis, encephalopathy)
	Cerebral artery thrombosis > vascular dementia
Depression	Psychosocial stress, disease process, iatrogenic (e.g. steroids)

• Psychosis due to lupus is uncommon. It usually occurs early in the disease and is associated with multisystem lupus activity.

Disorders of the basal ganglia

• Neural circuits linking the basal ganglia, frontal cortex and thalamus are involved in movement, attention, memory and reward processes. Basal ganglia disorders are characterised by movement, mental state and cognitive abnormalities.

Parkinson's disease

• Parkinson's disease (PD) affects over 1% of the population over 50 and results from deficient striatal dopaminergic activity.
• The table below shows the common psychiatric complications:
• The risk of dementia increases with age and duration of PD (78% after eight years). Symptoms are similar to those of dementia with Lewy bodies (Chapter 32). Coexistent Alzheimer's pathology is common.
• Cognitive deficits may be:
  • frontal lobe and other isolated focal abnormalities (e.g. memory, visuospatial difficulties) due to neurodegeneration

Table 29.3 Psychiatric complications of Parkinson's disease and their likely cause

	Prevalence	Cause
Depression and anxiety	40%	Disease process (dopaminergic, serotonergic, cholinergic limbic pathway dysfunction); psychosocial factors
Dementia	30%	Disease process
Other cognitive impairments	20%	Disease process, iatrogenic or related to depression
Psychosis	25%	Iatrogenic, disease process
Apathy	30%	Disease process
Impulsivity	<14%	Iatrogenic

Psychiatry at a Glance, Sixth Edition. Cornelius Katona, Claudia Cooper, Mary Robertson. © 2016 John Wiley & Sons, Ltd. Published 2016 by John Wiley & Sons, Ltd.
Companion website: www.ataglanceseries.com/psychiatry

- iatrogenic (e.g. antimuscarinic compounds and selegiline)
- related to depression.
- Psychosis most commonly presents with visual hallucinations and persecutory delusions and sometimes with pathological jealousy. It is more common in people with cognitive impairment and on increasing anti-Parkinsonian medication.
- Depression is associated with faster decline in cognitive function and activities of daily living and is a risk factor for dementia.
- A wide range of impulsive and compulsive behaviours, such as pathological gambling, hypersexuality, compulsive shopping and binge-eating, hypomania (in 2%) and euphoria (in 10%), are reported. They are almost always triggered by dopaminergic therapy.
- Treatment of depression and psychoses should be with drugs with a relatively low risk of extrapyramidal side effects (e.g. the antipsychotic quetiapine, the antidepressant citalopram).

Huntington's disease

- HD manifests at all ages, affects men and women equally, and prevalence is 4–7/100 000. It is characterised by cognitive decline, choreiform involuntary movements and personality change. Death usually occurs about 15 years after diagnosis.
- It is inherited as an autosomal dominant gene (100% penetrance) on chromosome 4. Rarely individuals have a negative family history, due to a new mutation or mistaken parentage. Recent findings suggest that the HD aetiology is more complex than originally thought. For example, the length of the CAG repeat is inversely correlated with age of onset, while both environmental and genetic factors can further modulate this parameter. An exciting recent study demonstrated that increased dosage of the glucose transporter gene SLC2A3 delayed the age at onset in HD, and this correlated with increased levels of the neuronal glucose transporter in HD patient cells.
- There is cerebral atrophy and reduced γ-aminobutyric acid (GABA), resulting in dopamine hypersensitivity.
- Cognitive impairments usually progress to subcortical dementia, with mental slowing, impaired executive functioning and a decline in memory; speech deteriorates faster than comprehension.
- Psychiatric disturbances are common in HD. Depression can also precede other symptoms.
- There is an increased risk of suicide in patients with HD and in those at risk (as high as 10%); this must be considered when planning predictive testing.
- Treatment is symptomatic, and depression and psychoses should be treated with standard medications. Atypical antipsychotics are preferred because they are less likely to exacerbate motor symptoms.

Hepatolenticular degeneration (Wilson's disease)

- This is a rare autosomal recessive disorder (chromosome 13).
- Excess copper deposition occurs in the lenticular nuclei. Timely treatment with penicillamine will usually reverse the neurologic symptoms and may ameliorate the psychiatric symptoms.
- Depression (20%), emotional lability, personality and behavioural changes (irritability, antisocial behaviour, disinhibition), poor school performance and alcohol abuse have been reported.

Table 29.4 Psychiatric complications of Huntington's disease and their likely cause

	Cause
Cognitive impairments that usually progress to subcortical dementia	Disease process
Irritability, aggression	Inability to communicate; executive dysfunction
Apathy (40–50%)	Iatrogenic, depression
Depression (40%)	Psychosocial stress; disease process (e.g. neuronal loss in the medial caudate, that connects to limbic structures)
Mania (10%) and psychosis (3–12%)	Disease process, e.g. dopaminergic excess

Sleep disorders

- **Narcolepsy** has a prevalence of 0.025%. The symptoms are:
  - excessive daytime sleepiness;
  - cataplexy (falling down suddenly after losing body tone, often in response to strong emotions);
  - sleep paralysis (paralysis on waking or going to sleep);
  - hypnogogic hallucinations.
- Stimulants such as methylphenidate and modafinil are used in treatment.
- **REM sleep behaviour disorder**: individuals act out their dreams, with associated risk of harm to themselves and others. Disturbances occur during REM sleep. The normal atonia of REM sleep is lost. It can be idiopathic or associated with PD, Lewy body dementia or Guillain-Barré syndrome. Treatment involves clonazepam and making the sleep environment safe.

Tic disorders

- Tics are very common, affecting 4–28% of young people. Possible diagnoses include:
  - transient tic disorder (tics lasting 1 year), (note: not included in DSM-5)
  - chronic vocal or chronic motor tic disorder (>1 year)
  - *Tourette's syndrome* (TS, multiple motor tics and one or more vocal/phonic tics for >1 year). In ICD 10 this is Gilles de la Tourette syndrome; in DSM-5 is Tourette's disorder.
- TS occurs in 1% of children aged 5–18 years. Males are more often affected (3–4:1).
- Recently it has been emphasised that there are many both neurological and psychiatric phenotypes: the only replicated phenotype is 'Pure TS' (tics only).
- The family history is frequently positive for tics, TS, obsessive-compulsive behaviour (OCB) and obsessive–compulsive disorder (OCD). No gene has been identified yet, but areas of interest have been demonstrated in some genetic studies (eg GWAS (Genome Wide Association Study).
- Both TS and tics are more common in people with learning disability and autistic spectrum disorders (ASD).
- Aetiology may include genetic vulnerability, pre- and perinatal problems (smoking, alcohol, cannabis, psychosocial stressors during pregnancy (may affect the severity/phenotype)): a suggestion of possibly infections (e.g. group A ß-haemolytic streptococcus), which gave rise to more plausible neuro-immunological

hypotheses, and androgens. Little is known about aetiology and phenotype.

- TS usually begins with facial tics such as excessive blinking; the median age at onset is 7 years. Vocal/phonic tics usually begin later. Tics can be simple (eye blinking, nose twitching, throat clearing, coughing) or complex (e.g. raspberries or twirling). Tics usually improve in severity by age 18 but are normally life-long (however, with reduced severity, distress, need for medication in adulthood). Associated symptoms include coprolalia (in 10% – involuntary swearing as a tic), copropraxia (involuntary rude sign as gesture), echolalia and echopraxia (copying what others say and do) and palilalia (repeating oneself), self-injurious behaviours and NOSI (non-obscene socially inappropriate behaviours, e.g. shouting 'Bomb' in an aeroplane/airport). TS is often comorbid with attention-deficit hyperactivity disorder (ADHD/Hyperkinetic Disorder), OCB/OCD and maybe ASD. There are many coexistent psychopathologies (e.g. depression, anxiety, phobias, personality disorder etc).

- Treatment is with:
  - psychoeducation for the patient and the family;
  - behavioural therapy, e.g. habit reversal training, CBIT (Comprehensive Behavioural Intervention for Tics);
  - medication: antipsychotics (for tics), clonidine with or without stimulants (e.g. atomoxetine) (for ADHD).

Note: We kept tic disorders in this section: in DSM-5 they are grouped under Neurodevelopmental Disorders (307.23) and further subdivided into Motor Disorders.

30 Neuropsychiatry III

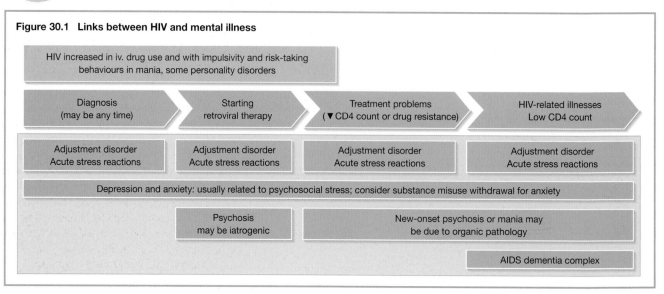

Figure 30.1 Links between HIV and mental illness

HIV increased in iv. drug use and with impulsivity and risk-taking behaviours in mania, some personality disorders

| Diagnosis (may be any time) | Starting retroviral therapy | Treatment problems (▼ CD4 count or drug resistance) | HIV-related illnesses Low CD4 count |

| Adjustment disorder Acute stress reactions | Adjustment disorder Acute stress reactions | Adjustment disorder Acute stress reactions | Adjustment disorder Acute stress reactions |

Depression and anxiety: usually related to psychosocial stress; consider substance misuse withdrawal for anxiety

| Psychosis may be iatrogenic | New-onset psychosis or mania may be due to organic pathology |

AIDS dementia complex

Infectious causes of neuropsychiatric symptoms

HIV and AIDS

- In the developed world, the prevalence of HIV is rising, in part because antiretroviral therapy prolongs life. In the UK there are around 7000 new diagnoses of HIV a year. In Western Europe, more than half of new diagnoses have been acquired through heterosexual contact, three-quarters in migrants or immigrants. Intravenous drug abusers remain a high-risk group, despite harm-reduction strategies.
- Regardless of treatment advances, HIV is still a stigmatising diagnosis in many sections of society.

The worried well

- People (not all of whom are at risk of HIV) may become pre-occupied with the possibility of becoming infected. Repeated requests for HIV serological testing may reflect:
  - depression or anxiety;
  - hypochondriacal disorder;
  - (more rarely) psychotic depression or schizophrenia, which may present with the delusion that the person is HIV-positive.

Psychological reactions to HIV infection

- Patients with HIV may undergo periods of crisis on first learning that they are infected, starting retroviral treatment, if tests indicate a problem with treatment (CD4 count falling or drug resistance) or when they first develop an HIV-related illness. They may react to these crises with:
  - acute stress reactions or adjustment disorders (see Chapter 10);
  - depression or anxiety;
  - deliberate self-harm – suicide is increased more than 20-fold in HIV-positive individuals.

Mental illness and HIV

- Drug and alcohol misuse are associated with both HIV and mental illness.

- HIV increases the likelihood of mental illness, and impulsive behaviour associated with some mental illnesses may increase the likelihood of infection (see Figure 30.1). There is therefore a sizeable population living with both HIV and psychiatric illness.
- Once infected, people with mental illness may be less likely to adhere to the complicated regimens of retroviral treatment.
- The patient's right to confidentiality may in rare cases need to be balanced against the need to protect others if health professionals become aware that the patient is putting others at risk (e.g. through unprotected sex).
- ***Depression*** is common at all stages of HIV and AIDS.
  - The diagnosis of depressive illness may be difficult. Apathy and fatigue may be due to retroviral therapy. Fatigue and weight loss may also be caused by declining CD4 counts and rising viral loads, so advancing HIV infection must be considered in the differential diagnosis.
  - AIDS-related dementia (now rare) may also present as a depression-like illness.
  - Anhedonia, hopelessness and suicidal thinking are likely to reflect true depressive illness.
  - Depression often reduces medication adherence and has been associated with an increase in CD4 count decline, so screening for it is an important part of HIV care.
  - Depression may worsen the disabling effects of AIDS.
- HIV-positive patients may also present with ***acute mania*** or ***schizophrenia-like psychoses***.
  - These may have been present before HIV diagnosis.
  - New onset cases are often associated with MRI/CT brain abnormalities, suggesting organic pathology.
- Caution is required when prescribing for HIV because of drug interactions and high sensitivity to side effects, especially extrapyramidal side effects.
- ***AIDS dementia complex*** occurs with a very low CD4 count (<200) and raised viral load. It is thought to be a direct manifestation of HIV infection within the brain, known as HIV-I

associated dementia. This has become rare in the developed world since the introduction of highly active antiretroviral therapy (HAART). Opportunistic infections such as parvovirus, *Toxoplasma gondii*, cryptococcal meningitis, neurosyphilis, tuberculous meningitis, cytomegalovirus encephalitis, increased vascular risk factors and tumours (e.g. lymphomas) can also contribute to a dementia syndrome.

Viral encephalitis

• The most common cause of viral encephalitis in the West is herpes simplex.
• Presentation is usually with severe headache, vomiting and reduced consciousness, but occasionally with psychosis, seizures or delirium.
• At least 50% of survivors experience disturbed behaviour, concentration or social adjustment, some with chronic cognitive impairment.

Syphilis

• One type of tertiary syphilis (symptoms that occur some years after infection, often a decade) is **general paralysis of the insane**. Symptoms include:
  • personality changes (disinhibition, irritability, lability);
  • cognitive changes (poor concentration);
  • dementia (20–40%);
  • depression (25%);
  • grandiosity (10%) and, more rarely, mania and schizophrenia-like psychoses.
• The main blood test for syphilis is VDRL. Intramuscular penicillin remains the first-line treatment.

Prion disease

• Human forms of *spongiform encephalopathy* (prion disorders, e.g. Creutzfeld–Jacob disease (CJD)) are rare (1/million per year) and are characterised by accumulation of an abnormal form of a normal host protease-resistant protein (PrP) in the brain.
• They present with a rapidly fatal dementia associated with myoclonic jerks.

• About 85% of cases are sporadic; the remaining cases of classical CJD are either familial (15%; sometimes autosomal dominant) or very rarely iatrogenic. A new form of CJD (variant CJD) was reported in younger adults (average age 27) in the UK in 1996 and appeared to relate to consumption of beef infected by bovine spongiform encephalopathy (BSE).
• Whereas classic CJD usually presents with physical symptoms, variant CJD most frequently starts with psychiatric symptoms (mood swings, fatigue, social withdrawal).

Metabolic disturbance

• *Acute intermittent porphyria* is the commonest type of porphyria (but still rare). Acute attacks occur spontaneously or may be precipitated by drugs (e.g. oral contraceptives, hypoglycaemics, alcohol), infections, pregnancy or low carbohydrate intake. Clinical presentation may be abdominal (colicky pain, vomiting, constipation) or neurological (peripheral neuropathy, bulbar palsies, epilepsy). Psychiatric disturbances include delirium (50%), depression, emotional lability and schizophrenia-like psychoses.

Endocrine

Table 30.1 lists some endocrine disorders and the psychiatric disorders they are associated with.

Nutritional disorders

• *Vitamin B₁₂* deficiency results in pernicious anaemia. This may be accompanied by subacute combined degeneration of the spinal cord, which is associated with signs of neuropathy and spinal cord involvement. Psychiatric symptoms include slowing of mental processes, confusion, memory problems, intellectual impairment, depression and paranoid delusions.
• Thiamine (B1) deficiency can result in Wernicke's encephalopathy and Korsakoff's psychosis (Chapter 18). In the developed world, this is most commonly associated with alcohol dependence.

Table 30.1 Psychiatric complications of endocrine disorders

Disorder	Depression/ anxiety	Behavioural disturbance	Psychosis	Cognitive changes
Hyperthyroidism	anxiety, depression	irritability; occasionally apathy and poor appetite in older people	psychotic depression reported	
Hypothyroidism *Hyperparathyroidism* *Primary hypoparathyroidism*	depression, anxiety depression	acute agitation apathy emotional lability	hallucinations occasionally reported after parathyroidectomy	dementia, delirium, occasionally memory deficits poor concentration, cognitive impairment, delirium after parathyroidectomy
Hypercortisolaemia: usually iatrogenic (steroids)	depression		mania	
Hypocortisolaemia (Addison's disease)	depression	apathy		
Hypopituitarism	depression	irritability		impaired memory
Phaeochromocytoma	episodic anxiety			

31 Acute Confusional States

- The acute confusional state (also known as delirium) is characterised by the rapid onset of a global but fluctuating dysfunction of the central nervous system (CNS) due to an underlying infectious, toxic, vascular, epileptic or metabolic cause.
- It may occur in as many as one-third of older patients admitted to hospital either at initial presentation or during hospitalisation.
- It represents one of the most important conditions encountered in liaison psychiatry and is seen by a wide range of specialities, including general and emergency medicine, general and orthopaedic surgery, and medicine for older people.
- It is associated with increased mortality and longer duration of hospitalisation.

Clinical features

- The DSM5 /ICD-10 diagnosis of delirium requires:

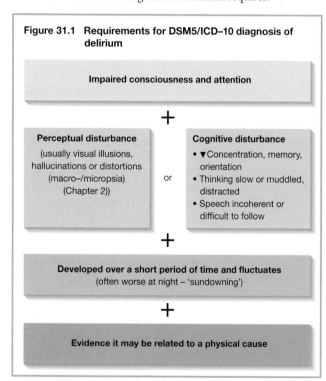

Figure 31.1 Requirements for DSM5/ICD–10 diagnosis of delirium

Impaired consciousness and attention

+

Perceptual disturbance
(usually visual illusions, hallucinations or distortions (macro–/micropsia) (Chapter 2))

or

Cognitive disturbance
- ▼Concentration, memory, orientation
- Thinking slow or muddled, distracted
- Speech incoherent or difficult to follow

+

Developed over a short period of time and fluctuates
(often worse at night – 'sundowning')

+

Evidence it may be related to a physical cause

- Based on the clinical presentation, delirium can be divided into two subtypes:
  - hypoactive – characterised by withdrawn, quiet, sleepy behaviour, is less likely to be recognised;
  - hyperactive – characterised by restless, agitated and aggressive behaviour.
- *Mood* and *affect* may fluctuate rapidly (lability) and be accompanied by irritability or perplexity; apathy and depression are also found.
- Poorly systematised, transient *delusions* are common. These may be secondary to abnormal perceptions and are often persecutory, with associated ideas of reference.
- Sweating, tachycardia and dilated pupils reflect underlying *autonomic overactivity*.

- There may be disturbance of the sleep/wake cycle (e.g. patients may be more alert during the evening and drowsy during the day).

Aetiology

- High-risk groups (who should be screened for delirium when admitted to hospital or care homes) include:
  - people aged 65 and over,
  - people with diffuse brain disease (dementia or Parkinson's disease),
  - people with a current hip fracture,
  - the severely ill.
- Breakdown of the blood–brain barrier, dopaminergic excess and hypercortisolaemia have all been implicated.
- Figure 31.2 shows possible precipitants of acute confusional states.

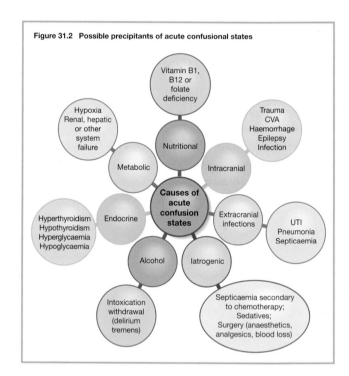

Figure 31.2 Possible precipitants of acute confusional states

Vitamin B1, B12 or folate deficiency

Hypoxia Renal, hepatic or other system failure

Trauma CVA Haemorrhage Epilepsy Infection

Nutritional

Metabolic

Intracranial

Hyperthyroidism Hypothyroidism Hyperglycaemia Hypoglycaemia

Endocrine

Causes of acute confusion states

Extracranial infections

UTI Pneumonia Septicaemia

Alcohol

Iatrogenic

Intoxication withdrawal (delirium tremens)

Septicaemia secondary to chemotherapy; Sedatives; Surgery (anaesthetics, analgesics, blood loss)

Differential diagnosis

- Delirium can be difficult to distinguish from dementia (Chapter 32) since people with established dementia are particularly vulnerable to delirium.
- The distinction from dementia with Lewy bodies, in which cognition typically fluctuates, may be particularly difficult.
- Other conditions that may resemble delirium are:
  - functional psychiatric conditions (mania, depression and late-onset schizophrenia);
  - responses to major stress, particularly severe pain;
  - dissociative disorders.

Here are some tips on telling delirium and dementia apart.

Psychiatry at a Glance, Sixth Edition. Cornelius Katona, Claudia Cooper, Mary Robertson. © 2016 John Wiley & Sons, Ltd. Published 2016 by John Wiley & Sons, Ltd.
Companion website: www.ataglanceseries.com/psychiatry

Table 31.1 Clinical features differentiating delirium and dementia

	Delirium	Dementia
Deterioration	Rapid (hours to days)	Slow (months to years)
Course	Fluctuating	Slowly progressive
Consciousness	Clouded	Alert
Thought content	Vivid, complex and muddled	Usually impoverished
Hallucinations	Very common and predominantly visual	In about a third; auditory or visual

- The diagnosis depends on:
  - the presence of the cardinal features of delirium (particularly fluctuation in both conscious level and cognitive impairment);
  - the presence of a specific underlying cause;
  - the lack of consistent features of affective or psychotic disorders.

Investigations

- It is imperative to obtain an informant history, focusing particularly on premorbid level of functioning, onset and course of the confusion, and use/abuse of drugs or alcohol.
- In the mental state assessment, particular attention should be paid to cognitive function (alertness, memory, language, visuospatial ability) and to fluctuation in behaviour.
- Physical examination is crucial in identifying focal neurological signs and evidence of infection or trauma.
- Appropriate blood investigations for confusion include:
  - full blood count (FBC) (to exclude anaemia, macrocytosis, leucocytosis);
  - erythrocyte sedimentation rate (ESR) (infection);
  - urea and electrolytes (U&E) (dehydration, electrolyte imbalance);
  - glucose;
  - thyroid function tests (TFT);
  - liver function tests (LFT);
  - calcium;
  - folate and B_{12};
  - VDRL (i.e. syphilis serology).
- Midstream urine (MSU) is mandatory.
- Chest x-ray (CXR) may be informative.
- Structural brain imaging (computed tomography (CT) or magnetic resonance imaging (MRI)) can identify many intracranial causes.
- Consider electroencephalography (EEG) if epilepsy is a differential.

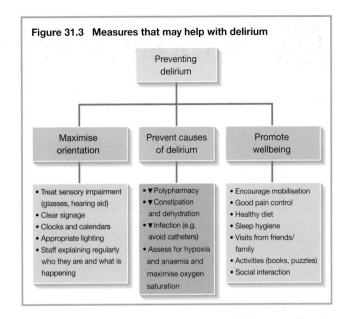

Figure 31.3 Measures that may help with delirium

Prevention

- Figure 31.3 shows measures that may help prevent delirium.

Management

- Specific management should be targeted at detection of the confusional state itself and at identification and subsequent treatment of underlying pathology. Patients should therefore usually be managed on general hospital (i.e. not psychiatric) wards.
- The preventative measures above are also good practice when treating delirium.
- If a person with delirium is distressed or considered a risk to him/herself or others and non-pharmacological measures are insufficient, medication may be needed.
  - Consider short-term (<1 week) antipsychotic (e.g. haloperidol, risperidone (not recommended in dementia)) or short-acting benzodiazepines (e.g. lorazepam).
  - Medication is preferable to physical restraint, but should be used sparingly.
  - Hypotensive and anticholinergic side effects may precipitate falls or exacerbate the confusion.
  - Longer acting benzodiazepines (e.g. diazepam or chlordiazepoxide) are used when the patient is withdrawing from alcohol or drug abuse.

Prognosis

- Delirium increases:
  - risk of dementia
  - mortality
  - length of stay of people already in hospital
  - risk of new admission to long-term care.

32 The Dementias

Definition and clinical presentation

- Dementia is a clinical syndrome rather than a diagnosis.
- It is acquired, progressive, usually irreversible global deterioration of higher cortical function in clear consciousness.
- Here are the diagnostic criteria and common symptoms:

Figure 32.1 Diagnostic criteria and common symptoms of dementia

Diagnosis requires:	Often present
Multiple cognitive deficits (e.g. memory, orientation, language, comprehension, reasoning, judgment)	**Behavioural problems** (e.g. apathy, aggression, wandering, restlessness, disinhibition, impulsivity)
+	**Depression and anxiety**
Resulting impairment in activities of daily living (e.g. washing, dressing, handling money)	**Psychotic symptoms** (in a 1/3) (e.g. persecutory delusions (aggravated by forgetfulness), visual and auditory hallucinations)
+	**Sleep problems** (e.g. insomnia, daytime drowsiness, confusion between day and night, nocturnal restlessness)
Clear consciousness	

- Presentation may occur months or years after the onset of symptoms and is often at family instigation because the person frequently has no insight into his or her deterioration. The clinical presentation may vary between different types of dementia.

Epidemiology

- Dementia is rare (<1%) before the age of 65 and becomes more common with increasing age. By the age of 90, the prevalence is 25%:

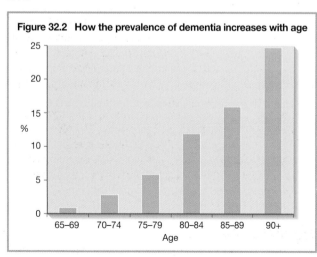

Figure 32.2 How the prevalence of dementia increases with age

- As the 'old' population in the developing world and the 'very old' population in the developed world increase, the number of people with dementia is projected to rise steeply.
- Low educational attainment, obesity, untreated systolic hypertension, depression and mental, social and physical inactivity increase the risk of late-life dementia.

Classification

- Here are the approximate prevalences of the most common types of dementia:

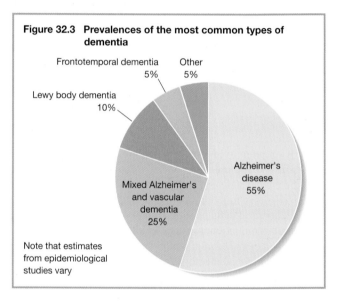

Figure 32.3 Prevalences of the most common types of dementia

Frontotemporal dementia 5%
Other 5%
Lewy body dementia 10%
Alzheimer's disease 55%
Mixed Alzheimer's and vascular dementia 25%

Note that estimates from epidemiological studies vary

- Dementias are sometimes classified as cortical or subcortical, although in reality pathology usually involves both cortical and subcortical tissue and the clinical features of both types overlap

Table 32.1 Cortical and subcortical dementias

	Cortical dementias	**Subcortical dementias**
Brain areas affected	cerebral cortex	basal ganglia, thalamus
Examples*	Alzheimer's disease, Lewy body dementia, frontotemporal dementia	Parkinson's disease dementia, Huntington's disease dementia, AIDS dementia, complex alcohol-related dementia
Typical symptoms	memory impairment, dysphasia, visuospatial impairment, problem-solving and reasoning deficits	psychomotor slowing, impaired memory retrieval, depression, apathy, executive dysfunction, personality change, language relatively preserved

*Vascular can be either, depending on the areas of brain affected.

Psychiatry at a Glance, Sixth Edition. Cornelius Katona, Claudia Cooper, Mary Robertson. © 2016 John Wiley & Sons, Ltd. Published 2016 by John Wiley & Sons, Ltd.
Companion website: www.ataglanceseries.com/psychiatry

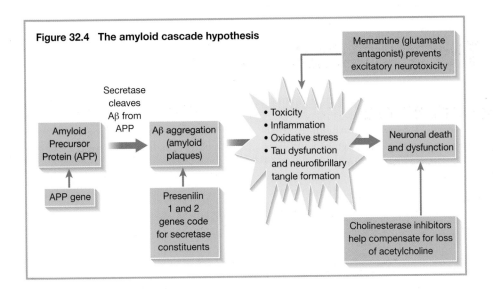

Figure 32.4 The amyloid cascade hypothesis

Alzheimer's disease

• The onset of Alzheimer's disease (AD) is gradual, usually with memory loss.

• Macroscopically, the brain is shrunken, with increased sulcal widening and enlarged ventricles.

• Microscopically, the key changes are neuronal loss and the presence (particularly in the cortex and the hippocampus) of **neurofibrillary tangles** and **amyloid plaques**. A protein called **Aβ** is the main constituent of amyloid plaques. It is cleaved from the **amyloid precursor protein (APP)** by a secretase enzyme. There is an association between dementia severity and the number of plaques in the brain. The **amyloid cascade hypothesis** states that AD is caused by an imbalance of (too much) brain Aβ production and (too little) Aβ clearance (see Figure 32.4).

• Mutations that increase the risk of AD have been identified in three genes: the APP gene and two genes coding for constituents of the secretase enzyme (**presenilin 1** and **presenilin 2**). These account for most cases of familial (early-onset) AD, in which inheritance is autosomal dominant.

• Inheritance of late-onset AD is multifactorial and polygenic, the **Apolipoprotein E (ApoE)** gene contributing most to the genetic aetiological component. Three common alleles of ApoE exist (E2, E3, E4); the E4 allele (particularly if homozygous) indicates increased risk and likelihood of earlier onset.

• Neurochemically, there are deficits in several neurotransmitters, particularly acetylcholine, noradrenaline, serotonin and somatostatin, with corresponding loss of the cell bodies of neurones secreting these transmitters.

Vascular dementia

• This is associated with more patchy cognitive impairment than AD; focal neurological symptoms or signs appear in a 'stepwise' rather than a continuous deterioration.

• Many people with dementia have a mixed picture of AD and vascular pathology, and patterns of progression differ less than previously thought between these dementias.

• Pathologically, there is at least one area of cortical infarction. There is a ninefold increase in risk of dementia in the year after a stroke. Vascular risk factors such as hypertension, hypercholesterolaemia, diabetes and smoking are risk factors for both vascular dementia and AD.

Dementia with Lewy bodies

• Dementia with Lewy bodies (DLB) is characterised by fluctuating cognition and alertness, vivid visual hallucinations, spontaneous Parkinsonism, sensitivity to neuroleptic medication and a sleep disorder. It is associated with the presence of Lewy bodies and neurites in the basal ganglia and cerebral cortex. Pathological changes characteristic of AD are also often found.

• A quarter of people with Parkinson's disease develop dementia, and 80% of patients with Parkinson's disease still alive after 20 years of follow-up develop dementia. Where Parkinson's disease predates the dementia by more than a year, the term 'Parkinson's disease dementia' (2–4% of all dementias) is used.

Frontotemporal dementia

• Frontotemporal dementia (FTD) has a younger mean age of onset and accounts for up to 20% of early-onset dementias but <10% of older onset. It is characterised by early personality changes and relative intellectual sparing. It mainly affects the frontal and anterior temporal lobes; pathology is heterogeneous with most cases having ubiquitin or tau positive inclusions.

Alcohol-related dementia

• This accounts for up to 10% of cases.

Normal pressure hydrocephalus

• This may be idiopathic or the result of subarachnoid haemorrhage, head injury or meningitis. It presents with marked mental slowness, apathy, wide-based gait and urinary incontinence. Ventriculoatrial shunting leads to frequent complications and tends to benefit only patients with prominent neurological signs and relatively mild dementia.

Dementia may occasionally be associated with repeated head trauma (e.g. boxers), subdural haematoma, Huntington's chorea, motor neurone disease (always FTD) or infection (e.g. HIV, syphilis, prion disease) (see Chapters 29–31). Dementias due to metabolic abnormalities (e.g. hyperparathyroidism, hypothyroidism) occur rarely.

Management

• Patients should have a full assessment to exclude treatable causes and identify specific problems (see Chapter 4 for risk management). The possibility of superimposed and treatable acute confusional states (commonly iatrogenic or secondary to infection) should be considered if a patient suddenly deteriorates.

• Depression sometimes precedes or complicates established dementia and has a poor response to antidepressants. Controlling vascular risk factors in patients with vascular dementia and prescribing low-dose aspirin reduce the risk of further stroke-related deterioration.

• Cholinesterase inhibitors (donepezil, rivastigmine, galantamine) can arrest or temporarily reverse cognitive and functional decline in people with mild to moderate AD and DLB, and may also improve behaviour.

• Memantine, which modulates glutamate neurotransmission, is used in moderate to severe AD.

• No currently available drugs can treat the underlying dementia, although these are targets of current research.

• Treatment of neuropsychiatric symptoms is important both for the patient's direct benefit and because they predict caregiver distress and breakdown of care.

• Careful risk assessment and management is critical (Chapter 4).

• Social support may include home care, day centres and intermittent respite organised by Social Services. Patients with severe dementia may require residential, nursing or continuing care (in hospital or other appropriate facility).

• Psychological techniques such as cognitive stimulation (group activities to actively stimulate and engage people with dementia) or teaching behavioural management techniques (see Glossary) to carers may improve cognition and behaviour.

Prognosis

• The gradient of cognitive decline is variable and depends on the type of dementia and age. People with dementia die earlier than others of the same age, even taking into account physical health. Premature death may occur before the dementia becomes severe.

• Those who progress to severe dementia usually need full nursing care; death is often from bronchopneumonia. Skilled nursing care has greatly increased life expectancy.

• Patients with vascular dementia have a slightly worse prognosis than those with AD; progression is less consistent with vulnerability to sudden cardiovascular or stroke-related death.

Cognitive impairment in people without dementia

• The term 'mild cognitive impairment' (MCI) is used to describe deterioration in cognition that is insufficient to meet criteria for dementia. Around 15% of people with MCI develop dementia within a year and about 50% within three years.

• In subjective cognitive impairment (SCI), people report cognitive problems (e.g. difficulties remembering names and where they put things) but perform within the normal range on psychometric tests for their age and education.

• A third of the general population report being forgetful and most will not progress to dementia, although there is growing evidence that MCI is preceded by around 15 years of SCI.

• Severe depression in old age may present with a 'pseudodementia' with prominent forgetfulness and poor self-care. Such patients usually have a short history and are often aware of, and distressed by, their poor function.

• Slowly progressive acute confusional states (e.g. subdural haematoma, myxoedema and vitamin deficiencies) may present with a dementia-like picture.

Psychiatric Management   Part 6

33 Psychological Therapies

Figure 33.1 The three areas of psychological therapy

Supportive therapies
- Usually unstructured
- Duration varies but often 6–10 sessions establishing rapport, facilitating emotional expression, reflection, reassurance
- Non-directive problem-solving, e.g. for adjustment disorders, stress, bereavement
- Mild depression or anxiety

Cognitive and behavioural therapies
- Structured focus on what client wants to change in life
- Explicit – gives client clear strategies
- Time limited, typically 6–12 sessions
- Cognitive: identify automatic negative thoughts and core beliefs
- Behavioural graded exposure
- Activity scheduling
- **A**ntecedents **B**ehaviour **C**onsequences (**ABC**), e.g. for
  - depression, anxiety
  - eating disorders
  - personality disorders
  - psychotic disorders

Psychodynamic therapies
- Unstructured
- Often for years
- Free association (client talks about what comes to mind and therapist interprets this)
- Transference
- Counter-transference, e.g. for
  - personality disorders
  - longstanding depression or anxiety

Counselling/ supportive psychotherapy

Cognitive behavioural therapy (CBT)

Behavioural therapies Behavioural activation Behavioural management therapy

Psychoanalysis 4–5x week for years

Therapeutic communities

Psychodynamic psychotherapy 1–2x week for >year

Newer therapies

Based on CBT →

Dialectical behavioural therapy (DBT) Lasts about a year Group and individual sessions for borderline personality disorder

Based on psychodynamic and CBT therapies →

Eye movement desensitisation and reprocessing therapy (EMDR)

Based on psychodynamic psychotherapy →

Interpersonal therapy (IPT)

Mentalisation based therapy For borderline personality disorder

---

How therapies work

- Psychological therapies work by helping people understand why they feel as they do. They can do this by:
  - reflecting with clients about how past and present life events have affected their relationship styles and patterns of thinking, and how these might affect their current mental state;
  - using the client–therapist relationship as a tool (e.g. modeling good communication, exploring how emotions felt towards the therapist might reflect those in other relationships);
  - teaching skills (e.g. problem-solving, communication).
- The therapist can support the clients to change the way they interact and perceive the world, to come to terms with past stresses and cope more effectively with current and future stresses.

Types of therapy (see Figure 33.1)

- There are three broad categories of psychological therapy:
  - supportive therapies
  - cognitive and behavioural therapies
  - psychodynamic psychotherapies.
- More recently designed therapies have been based on the principles of these therapies.
- Choice of therapy will be guided by patient preference, illness characteristics and cost-effectiveness. Treatments may involve individual, group, couple or family interventions.
- Group therapy emphasises interrelationships within the group where problems are shared.
- Family therapy may be systemic or behavioural. Systemic theory assumes that problems have arisen with the 'system' of family

Psychiatry at a Glance, Sixth Edition. Cornelius Katona, Claudia Cooper, Mary Robertson. © 2016 John Wiley & Sons, Ltd. Published 2016 by John Wiley & Sons, Ltd.
Companion website: www.ataglanceseries.com/psychiatry

functioning, not just the individual. It is used predominantly in child and adolescent psychiatry. The expectation is that improved family functioning will result in improvement in the patient.

Cognitive behavioural therapy (CBT)

- Some people hold unhelpful core beliefs or 'silent assumptions' that they learn from early, traumatic life experiences.
- These people are more vulnerable to depression. When exposed to stress at a later date, these core beliefs are activated and they have **negative automatic thoughts**.
- These negatively biased thoughts play a role in the persistence of depression because they sustain the underlying negative beliefs in the face of contrary evidence.

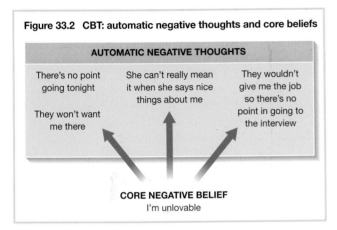

Figure 33.2 CBT: automatic negative thoughts and core beliefs

- The aim of CBT is initially to help individuals to identify and challenge these automatic negative thoughts and then to modify any abnormal underlying core beliefs. The latter is important in reducing the risk of relapse.
- CBT is used to treat depression, anxiety, eating disorders and some personality disorders. It can also be used to treat psychosis (see Chapter 7).

CBT case example: A woman who complains that she has no friends discovers during CBT that she has a tendency to jump to the conclusion that people find her boring. She developed this habit in childhood because her mother consistently ignored or rejected her. Together with her therapist she plans an 'experiment' to initiate a conversation with a colleague at work. The colleague responds positively and in the next session she realises that she has automatic negative thoughts that she is boring and she starts to challenge these.

Behavioural therapies

- These are based on learning theory. Operant conditioning encourages desirable behaviours by positive reinforcement and discourages undesirable behaviours by withholding reinforcement (negative reinforcement).
- Avoiding feared items, places or actions increases the anxiety associated with them. If people challenge their avoidance, their anxiety will rise but then eventually decrease (**habituation**). Techniques include graded exposure to a hierarchy of anxiety-producing situations (systematic desensitisation) – for example, to a spider in a glass box, then one on the other side of the room, finally on the patient's hand. In flooding, the patient is rapidly exposed to an anxiety-producing stimulus. Reciprocal inhibition couples the desensitisation with a response incompatible with the symptom. For example, habit reversal training, used in Tourette's syndrome, aims to increase awareness of tics, training to develop a competing

response and social support from an identified person (example partner, parent). A competing response involves selection and implementation of a physically incompatible behaviour to prevent tics or make them more difficult: for example for a lateral head jerking tic could be to tense the neck muscles (thus preventing the tic).

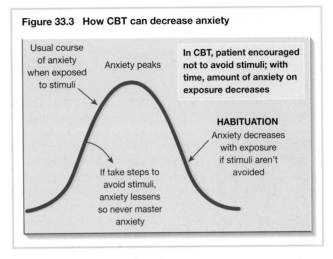

Figure 33.3 How CBT can decrease anxiety

- **Behavioural activation** focuses on activity scheduling to encourage patients to approach activities that they are avoiding.
- **Behavioural management therapy** uses the 'ABC' approach, where observations are made on **A**ntecedents to target behaviour, the **B**ehaviour itself and its **C**onsequences. The antecedents and consequences can then be manipulated to increase or decrease the target behaviour as required. An example target behaviour may be aggression or wandering in dementia. Behavioural techniques are included in interpersonal psychotherapy, CBT and dialectical behaviour therapy (see below).
- **Behavioural couples therapy** is recommended for treatment of depression and anxiety in people who have a regular partner and where the relationship may contribute to the development or maintenance of depression.

Psychodynamic therapies

- Psychodynamic therapy is unstructured. It helps many who have longstanding personality disorders or undifferentiated psychological problems or for whom anxiety and/or depression are ingrained within a person's personality. It is based on psychoanalytic principles.
- Psychoanalysis stems from the work of Sigmund Freud. It views human behaviour as determined by unconscious forces derived from primitive emotional needs. Therapy aims to resolve longstanding underlying conflicts and unconscious defence mechanisms (e.g. denial, repression).
- Psychoanalysis explores the unconscious using free association (the patient saying whatever enters their mind) and the therapist interprets these statements. These interpretations make links between events in the patient's past experiences, current life and relationship with the therapist.
- Key therapeutic tools are:
  - **transference**: the patient re-experiences strong emotions from early important relationships in their relationship with the therapist;
  - **counter-transference**: the therapist experiences strong emotions towards the patient.
- In psychoanalysis, sessions are four to five times a week for 50 minutes for two to five years. **Psychodynamic psychotherapy** has the same theoretical basis as psychoanalysis but treatment sessions are less frequent (one to two times a week).

- **Therapeutic communities** are inpatient facilities run along psychodynamic lines and most frequently used to treat severe borderline personality disorder that has not responded to other therapies. Treatment involves group and individual sessions.

Newer therapies

- **Interpersonal psychotherapy (IPT)** is used to treat depression and eating disorders. It focuses on interpersonal aspects of the illness. All close relationships are carefully discussed, and any problems are conceptualised as difficulties in role transitions (e.g. promotion, loss of job, becoming a parent), interpersonal disputes, deficits in the number or quality of relationships, or grief. This formulation is the focus of discussion in subsequent sessions.
- **Dialectical behaviour therapy (DBT)** is designed for individuals with borderline personality disorder and is particularly intended to address their repeated self-harm behaviours. The therapy incorporates some components similar to CBT and also provides group skills training to equip the individual with alternative coping strategies (rather than deliberate self-harm) when faced with difficult problems or emotional instability. The skills taught include mindfulness (bringing one's attention back to the present moment), which is derived from Buddhist meditation.
- **Mentalisation-based treatments**, developed for people with borderline personality disorder, are based on psychodynamic principles and promote understanding in personal relationships by improving patients' ability to deduce the mental states that lie behind their own and other people's behaviour.
- **Eye movement desensitisation and reprocessing (EMDR)** is a psychotherapy treatment that aims to help patients access and process traumatic memories with the goal of emotionally resolving them. Clients recall emotionally disturbing material while simultaneously focusing on an external stimulus. This stimulus usually involves the therapist directing the patients' lateral eye movements by asking them to look first one way then the other (saccadic eye movements). It is an effective treatment for post-traumatic stress disorder (PTSD).

Improving access to psychological therapies (IAPT)

- Since 2006, the NHS IAPT programme has increased availability of brief psychological therapies for depression and anxiety in primary care in the UK.
- IAPT provides treatments recommended by NICE (National Institute for Health and Clinical Excellence). These are:
  - CBT for depression and anxiety disorders, including obsessive–compulsive disorder and PTSD
  - IPT, behavioural activation, counselling or couples therapy for depression
  - EMDR for PTSD.

34 Antipsychotics

Types of antipsychotic

- The first antipsychotic, chlorpromazine, was introduced in 1951 for anaesthetic (antiemetic) premedication. It was noted to reduce delusions and hallucinations in schizophrenia without causing excessive sedation.
- Antipsychotics are divided into typical (first-generation) and atypical (second-generation) drugs (see Table 34.1).
  - Typical antipsychotics are more likely to cause extrapyramidal side effects (EPSE), hyperprolactinaemia and tardive dyskinesia.
  - Atypical antipsychotics may be slightly better at treating negative symptoms of schizophrenia.
- Atypical antipsychotics are now recommended for first-line treatment of new onset psychosis, but typical antipsychotics are still used.

Table 34.1 Atypical and typical antipsychotics

Atypical antipsychotics	Typical antipsychotics	
clozapine	phenothiazines	chlorpromazine
risperidone		fluphenazine
quetiapine		trifluoperazine
olanzapine	butyrophenones	haloperidol
aripiprazole	thioxanthenes	flupentixol,
ziprasidone		zuclopenthixol
amisulpride	diphenylbutylpiperidines	pimozide
paliperidone	substituted benzamides	sulpiride

Clozapine

- Only clozapine has demonstrated superior efficacy to other antipsychotics. It substantially reduces overall mortality from schizophrenia because of a reduction in the rate of suicide.
- Because of potentially dangerous side effects, it is only prescribed if two different antipsychotics have failed to control symptoms.
- It may cause potentially fatal agranulocytosis (risk of death 1:10 000 exposed), and requires regular haematological monitoring (full blood count (FBC) once a week for 18 weeks, then fortnightly for a year, then monthly).
- There is also a risk of seizures.
- The most common side effects are listed in Figure 34.2. Associations with venous thromboembolism, myocarditis and cardiomyopathy have also been suggested.

How do antipsychotics work?

- Figure 34.1 shows the action of antipsychotics on brain neuroreceptors:
- We do not know exactly how these actions treat psychosis.
- Abnormal dopamine transmission can result in a false sense of having seen or heard something before, or of not having done so, leading to the experience of psychosis. It is thought that antipsychotics improve psychosis by diminishing this abnormal transmission by blocking the dopamine D2/3 receptors. Several brain regions may be involved, but the ventral striatum may have a critical role.

Figure 34.1 Actions of antipsychotics at brain receptors

Dopamine (D_2/D_3)	All antipsychotics reduce transmission. Almost all are antagonists. Aripiprazole is a partial D_2 agonist; full binding decreases dopamine availability by 30%. Typicals usually have higher affinity than atypicals
$5HT_{2a}$	Most atypical antipsychotics are potent antagonists
Cholinergic / Adrenergic / Histaminergic	Typical antipsychotics are potent antagonists

Mode of administration

- This is usually by mouth, sometimes with extensive 'first-pass' metabolism in the liver.
- Many can also be given by short-acting intramuscular (IM) or (very rarely) intravenous injection.
- Some (such as flupenthixol (Depixol), fluphenazine (Modecate) and risperidone (Risperdal)) can be given by depot injection every one to four weeks. This bypasses first-pass metabolism; it may improve adherence or at least allow closer monitoring.

Indications

- Treatment and relapse prevention in **schizophrenia and other psychoses** (e.g. mania, psychotic depression); they are most effective in alleviating positive symptoms such as delusions, hallucinations and thought disorder.
- Some atypical antipsychotics (risperidone, olanzapine and quetiapine) are licensed for treatment of **acute mania**.
- They are also used for treatment of **violent or agitated behaviour** (usually on inpatient wards) that does not respond to de-escalation. Haloperidol is most commonly used in this context, usually with a benzodiazepine.
- They are no longer recommended for treatment of behavioural disturbance in older people with dementia because of increased risk of stroke and impairment of glycaemic control, with the exception that risperidone is licensed for short-term use (up to six weeks) in this context.

Psychiatry at a Glance, Sixth Edition. Cornelius Katona, Claudia Cooper, Mary Robertson. © 2016 John Wiley & Sons, Ltd. Published 2016 by John Wiley & Sons, Ltd.
Companion website: www.ataglanceseries.com/psychiatry

Figure 34.2 Side effects of antipsychotics

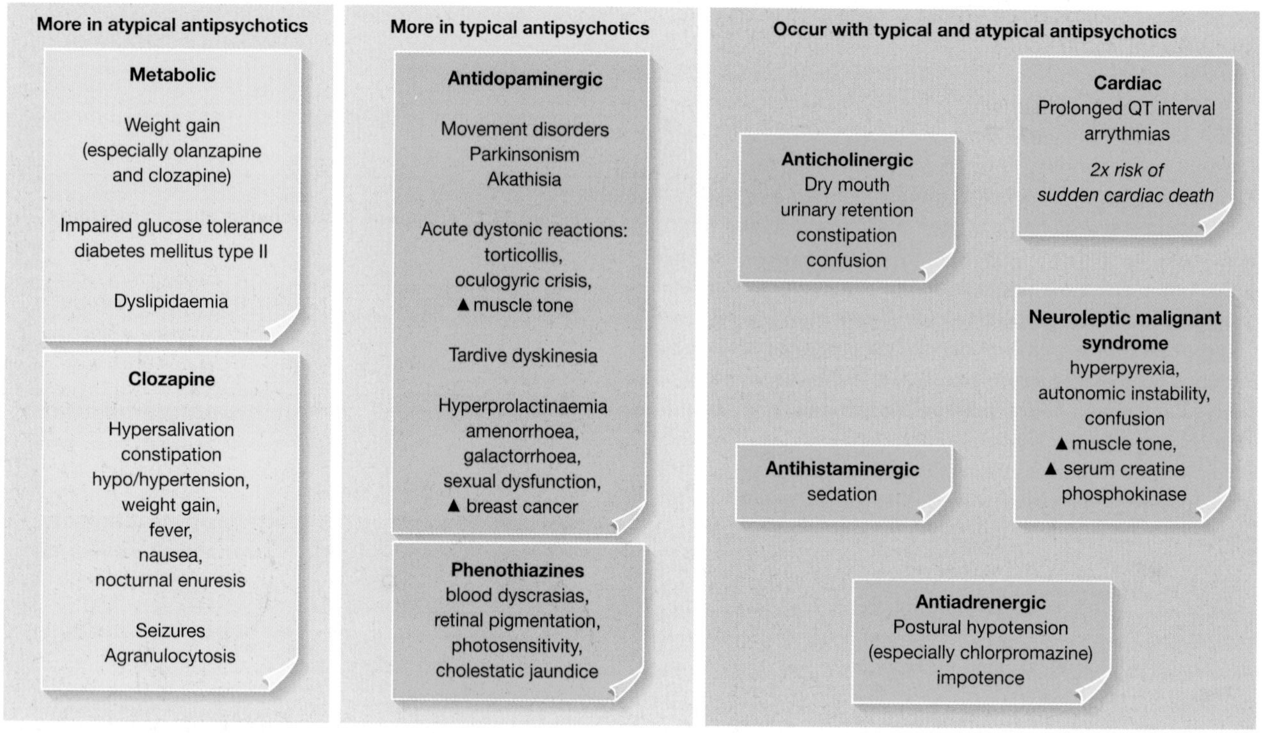

| More in atypical antipsychotics | More in typical antipsychotics | Occur with typical and atypical antipsychotics |

More in atypical antipsychotics

Metabolic

Weight gain
(especially olanzapine
and clozapine)

Impaired glucose tolerance
diabetes mellitus type II

Dyslipidaemia

Clozapine

Hypersalivation
constipation
hypo/hypertension,
weight gain,
fever,
nausea,
nocturnal enuresis

Seizures
Agranulocytosis

More in typical antipsychotics

Antidopaminergic

Movement disorders
Parkinsonism
Akathisia

Acute dystonic reactions:
torticollis,
oculogyric crisis,
▲ muscle tone

Tardive dyskinesia

Hyperprolactinaemia
amenorrhoea,
galactorrhoea,
sexual dysfunction,
▲ breast cancer

Phenothiazines
blood dyscrasias,
retinal pigmentation,
photosensitivity,
cholestatic jaundice

Occur with typical and atypical antipsychotics

Anticholinergic
Dry mouth
urinary retention
constipation
confusion

Cardiac
Prolonged QT interval
arrythmias

*2x risk of
sudden cardiac death*

**Neuroleptic malignant
syndrome**
hyperpyrexia,
autonomic instability,
confusion
▲ muscle tone,
▲ serum creatine
phosphokinase

Antihistaminergic
sedation

Antiadrenergic
Postural hypotension
(especially chlorpromazine)
impotence

- Antipsychotics are also used to treat **Tourette's syndrome** but generally in much lower doses than for the psychoses (e.g. haloperidol up to 5 mg/day); aripiprazole usually maximum 5–10 mgm/day.

Side effects

- Patients report that movement disorders, sedation, weight gain and sexual dysfunction are the most troublesome sideeffects.
- Because of their more potent dopaminergic effects, typical antipsychotics are more likely than atypical antipsychotics to cause:
  - **extrapyramidal movement disorders** (due to dopamine blockade in the nigrostriatal pathways):
    - Acute dystonia and Parkinsonism reflect drug-induced dopamine/acetylcholine imbalance and respond to anticholinergic drugs such as procyclidine.
    - Akathisia (psychomotor restlessness) is less responsive to anticholinergics; beta-blockers or benzodiazepines may be helpful.
    - Tardive dyskinesia is usually caused by long-term antipsychotics, thought to be because of dopamine-receptor supersensitivity and characterised by abnormal buccolingual masticatory movements and, in severe cases, choreiform trunk and limb movements, especially in older people. Reduction or cessation of anticholinergics (which do not help and may make it worse) and typical antipsychotics where possible and substitution of an atypical antipsychotic are recommended, although the condition

is irreversible in 50% of cases. Clozapine may treat the tardive dyskinesia as well as psychosis.
  - **raised prolactin** leading to endocrine effects (due to tuberoinfundibular pathway dopamine blockade).
- Atypical antipsychotics cause more **metabolic side effects**. Increased insulin resistance is the most likely cause.

Stopping antipsychotics

- It is generally recommended that antipsychotics should be continued for at least one to two years after a first episode of psychosis. As 98% of those discontinuing medication after two years relapse, many recommend that they are continued for five years.
- In practice, patients often discontinue antipsychotic medication long before this, with a quarter non-adherent 10 days post-discharge in one study.
- Patients should be advised to taper their medication over at least three weeks if they decide to stop because stopping suddenly doubles the risk of relapse.

Physical health monitoring

- Prior to commencing antipsychotics (and yearly thereafter), the following monitoring is recommended:
  - Body Mass Index and waist circumference;
  - ECG;
  - Blood tests: FBC, urea and electrolytes, blood lipids, liver function tests, glucose and HBA$_{1C}$, prolactin.

35 Antidepressants

Figure 35.1 The main groups of antidepressants and their side effects

Antidepressant	Side effects	
Serotonin–noradrenergic reuptake inhibitors • Fluoxetine • Citalopram • Paroxetine • Sertraline • Fluvoxamine	• Headache • Anorexia • Nausea • Indigestion • Anxiety • Sexual dysfunction ⚠ – ↑ suicide ideation; not recommended < 18 years (except fluoxetine) ⚠ – withdrawal syndrome	Selective serotonin reuptake inhibitors mainly: ⚠ • Gastrointestinal bleeding • Hyponatraemia in older people
Serotonin–noradrenergic reuptake inhibitors • Venlafaxine • Duloxetine		Venlafaxine: • Hypertension/hypotension • Cardiotoxic in overdose
Noradrenergic and specific serotonergic antidepressant • Mirtazapine	Dry mouth, drowsiness and weight gain	
Tricyclic antidepressants • Amitriptyline • Dothiepin • Imipramine • Lofepramine	• Anticholinergic • Antiadrenergic ⚠ – cardiac arrhythmias ⚠ – seizures	
Monoamine oxidase inhibitors • Phenelzine • Tranylcypromine	• Anticholinergic • Antiadrenergic • Tyramine reaction	
Melatonergic agonist • Agomelatine	• Nausea, diarrhoea, constipation, abdominal pain • Increased serum transaminases – headache, dizziness, drowsiness – anxiety, insomnia, fatigue – back pain – sweating	

• Selective serotonin reuptake inhibitors (SSRIs) (**citalopram, fluvoxamine, fluoxetine, sertraline** and **paroxetine**) were introduced in the 1980s and are now the most commonly prescribed class of antidepressants in the developed world.

• **Venlafaxine** and **duloxetine** are selective serotonin and noradrenaline reuptake inhibitors (SNRIs]).

• **Mirtazapine and mianserin** have a noradrenergic and selective serotonergic action.

• **Reboxetine** is a noradrenaline selective reuptake inhibitor.

• **Moclobemide** is a reversible inhibitor of MAO-A.

• **Agomelatine** is a melatonergic agonist and 5-HT antagonist.

• **Vortioxetine** has recently been licensed and affects serotonergic neurotransmission through multiple mechanisms.

• Other antidepressants available include **trazodone, maprotiline**, and **nefazodone**.

• The herbal preparation hypericum (St John's Wort), whose active ingredient is thought to be hypericin, is widely used and may be effective in mild to moderate depression. Its action is similar to that of monoamine oxidase inhibitors (MAOIs) and it may interact adversely with many other drugs.

• Antidepressants available prior to 1980 were divided into the tricyclics (such as **imipramine, amitriptyline, dothiepin** and **lofepramine**) and the MAOIs such as **phenelzine** and **tranylcypromine**. Tricyclic antidepressants are still in regular use, while MAOIs are occasionally prescribed.

How they work (see Figure 35.1)

• The common mechanism of action of antidepressants involves increasing neural transmission of monoamines (serotonin, noradrenaline and in some cases dopamine).

• The SSRIs and SNRIs do this by inhibiting their reuptake from the synaptic cleft.

• MAOIs inhibit the breakdown of serotonin (and to a lesser extent noradrenaline) at the synapse by inhibition of MAO-A.

• Mianserin and mirtazapine block presynaptic α_2-receptors. These are autoreceptors that usually inhibit neurotransmission as a negative feedback mechanism. Blocking α_2-receptors increases monamine output.

Psychiatry at a Glance, Sixth Edition. Cornelius Katona, Claudia Cooper, Mary Robertson. © 2016 John Wiley & Sons, Ltd. Published 2016 by John Wiley & Sons, Ltd.
Companion website: www.ataglanceseries.com/psychiatry

- When the monoamines bind to post-synaptic receptors, second messengers are released that result in increased production of transcription factors that control gene expression.
- These appear to increase production of Brain Derived Neurotrophic Factors (BDNF). The transcription factors are down-regulated by increased levels of cortisol (produced at times of stress).
- While the increase in monoamine availability in the synaptic cleft occurs within hours of taking antidepressants, antidepressants take around four weeks to show most of their effects clinically. The reasons for this are not certain: explanations include.
  - Four weeks may be the time it takes BDNF to increase neuroplasticity and neurogenesis in the hippocampus, reversing the atrophy of hippocampal neurons that results from depression.
  - The receptor sensitivity hypothesis has also been suggested to explain the delayed action of antidepressants. This proposes that depression results from supersensitivity and up-regulation of post-synaptic receptors that have too little stimulation. Increased availability of these neurotransmitters results in desensitisation and possibly a decrease in the number of receptors, and according to this theory it is this that lifts the patient's mood.

Indications

- The main indication for antidepressants is a moderate or severe depressive episode. They are not generally recommended for mild depression, for which active monitoring, problem-solving and exercise are preferred.
- They should be taken for at least four to six months after resolution of symptoms. Studies suggest a response rate of 60–70% (compared with 30% with placebo).
- Antidepressants are also useful in phobic anxiety, panic disorder, post-traumatic stress disorder (PTSD), general anxiety disorder (GAD), bulimia nervosa and obsessive–compulsive disorder (OCD) and in preventing depressive relapse. Bulimia and OCD often require higher doses (e.g. 60 mg fluoxetine).
- Buproprion is a dopamine and noradrenaline reuptake inhibitor that is commonly prescribed as an antidepressant in the USA. In the UK it is only licensed as a smoking cessation drug.

Mode of administration

- Antidepressants are taken orally. Most can be given once daily and are extensively and variably metabolised by first pass in the liver.
- The antidepressant response seldom occurs in less than two weeks and often not for four weeks, though early partial response is predictive of remission. Patients not warned of the delayed therapeutic action are likely to be less treatment adherent.

Side effects

- The main side effects of the most commonly prescribed antidepressants are listed in the table (see Figure 35.1).
- Tricyclic antidepressants may increase mortality from cardiovascular disease and are often fatally toxic in overdose. SSRIs display minimal cardiotoxicity even in overdose.
- SSRIs inhibit platelet aggregation and have been associated with an increased risk of gastrointestinal bleeding especially in older people, so should be avoided if possible in patients aged over 80 years, those with prior upper GI bleeding, or in those also taking aspirin or a non-steroidal anti-inflammatory drug.
- SSRIs may cause hyponatraemia in older people.
- There is evidence that SSRIs and SNRIs may increase agitation during the first one to two weeks of use. There have been some reports that SSRIs and venlafaxine may be associated with increased suicidal ideation and aggression, and because of these concerns all except fluoxetine are contraindicated in children under 18.
- Venlafaxine may cause hypertension (or hypotension).
- MAOIs can cause an occasionally fatal syndrome of hypertension and throbbing headache if foods containing large quantities of tyramine (e.g. cheese, red wine) are eaten.

Stopping antidepressants

- All antidepressants have the potential to cause withdrawal phenomena. They should not be stopped abruptly unless a serious adverse event has occurred. Gradual tapering over two to four weeks is recommended.
- Discontinuation symptoms include electric shock sensations, dizziness, increased mood change, restlessness, difficulty sleeping, unsteadiness, sweating, abdominal symptoms and altered sensations.

Serotonin syndrome

- Drugs that increase serotonin availability may cause serotonin syndrome. This is more likely where two such drugs are given in combination. Features of serotonin syndrome include confusion, delirium, shivering, sweating, changes in blood pressure and myoclonus.

Antidepressants in children

In 2003, following concerns that SSRIs may increase the risk of suicidal thoughts and self-harm, the Committee on Safety of Medicines recommended that fluoxetine was the only SSRI with a favourable balance of risks and benefits for use in the treatment for major depressive episode in young people under the age of 18. Other antidepressants are sometimes used by experts.

36 Other Psychotropic Drugs

Antimanic drugs (mood stabilisers)
Lithium
- Lithium is used for:
  - prophylaxis in recurrent affective disorder (unipolar and bipolar),
  - acute treatment of mania,
  - augmentation of antidepressants in resistant depression,
  - schizoaffective illness,
  - the control of aggression.
- We do not know the exact mechanism of action. We do know that:
  - lithium interacts with all biological systems where sodium, potassium, calcium or magnesium are involved;
  - at therapeutic blood levels it probably has effects on neurotransmission including 5HT, noradrenaline, dopamine and acetylcholine;
  - its interference with cyclic adenosine monophosphate (cAMP)-linked receptors explains its action on the thyroid and kidney.
- It is taken orally and excreted by the kidneys. It has a narrow therapeutic range (0.4–1.0 mmol/L). Monitoring should include:
  - **thyroid** and **renal** function prior to starting lithium and every six months while taking it;
  - serum **lithium levels** (initially weekly, thereafter every 12 weeks), blood being taken around 12 hours after the last dose.

Figure 36.1 Effects of lithium dosages

Below 0.4 mmol/L	0.4–1.0 mmol/L	Above 1.0 mmol/L
Ineffective	Therapeutic window	Toxic dose
	Side effects • Nausea • Fine tremor • Weight gain • Oedema • Polydipsia and polyuria • Exacerbation of psoriasis and acne • Hypothyroidism	**Signs of toxicity** • Vomiting • Diarrhoea • Coarse tremor • Slurred speech • Ataxia • Drowsiness and confusion • Convulsions and coma

- Treatment of toxicity or overdose involves cessation of lithium and fluid therapy to restore glomerular filtration rate (GFR), normalise urine output, and enhance lithium clearance.
- Contraindications: lithium should be avoided in renal, cardiac, thyroid and Addison's disease.
- Dehydration and diuretics can lead to lithium toxicity.
- Adverse interactions can also occur between lithium and non-steroidal anti-inflammatory drugs, calcium channel blockers and some antibiotics.

Other antimanic drugs
- Valproic acid (sodium valproate) and carbemazepine are also used for prophylaxis in bipolar disorder. Lamotrigine may be particularly effective in preventing depressive episodes. Here are their main side effects.

Table 36.1 Side effects of lamotrigine and valproic acid

Lamotrigine*	Valproic acid
skin reactions (including Stevens–Johnson syndrome)	nausea
aseptic meningitis drowsiness	gastric irritation
dizziness	diarrhoea
diplopia	weight gain
leucopenia insomnia nausea	

*May affect metabolism of other drugs including oral contraceptives, necessitating other contraceptive precautions.

Lithium, lamotrigine and valproic acid are teratogenic and should be avoided during pregnancy (especially first trimester) and lactation.

Hypnotics and anxiolytics
- The most commonly used are the benzodiazepines and zopiclone and related compounds.
- Benzodiazepines are anxiolytic, sleep inducing, anticonvulsant and muscle relaxant. Their indications include:
  - insomnia,
  - short-term (two to four weeks) use in generalised anxiety (but not phobia or panic disorder),
  - alcohol withdrawal states,
  - the control of violent behaviour.
- Underlying conditions (such as depression) should always be excluded and behavioural alternative treatments considered. Benzodiazepines are also used as 'second-line' drugs in refractory epilepsy.
- Zopiclone and zolpidem are commonly used hypnotics without anticonvulsant or muscle-relaxing properties.
- Antihistamines such as promethazine are available over the counter in Britain.
- Buspirone is licensed for short-term treatment of anxiety.

Mode of administration
- Usually administered orally.
- Intramuscular, intravenous and rectal benzodiazepines preparations are available and may be required in status epilepticus and violent patients.

Psychiatry at a Glance, Sixth Edition. Cornelius Katona, Claudia Cooper, Mary Robertson. © 2016 John Wiley & Sons, Ltd. Published 2016 by John Wiley & Sons, Ltd.
Companion website: www.ataglanceseries.com/psychiatry

Pharmacokinetics

- Most have active metabolites, some with half-lives of several days.
- The long-acting benzodiazepines include diazepam, chlordiazepoxide and nitrazepam.
- Lorazepam, oxazepam and temazepam are shorter acting benzodiazepines.

Mechanism of action

- Benzodiazepines, zopiclone and zolpidem potentiate the inhibitory effects of γ-aminobutyric acid (GABA).
- Buspirone is a 5HT1a partial agonist.

Side effects

- These include:
  - drowsiness and lightheadedness the next day,
  - ataxia (risk of falls in older people),
  - amnesia,
  - dependence,
  - disinhibition, which may lead (paradoxically) to aggression.
- Benzodiazepines potentiate alcohol and other sedatives; the combination is dangerous in overdose.

Overdose of benzodiazepines

Signs include respiratory depression, drowsiness, dysarthria and ataxia. Emergency treatment is with flumazenil, a selective benzodiazepine antagonist, although this can be hazardous in mixed overdoses (including tricyclic antidepressants) or in benzodiazepine-dependent patients, so should only be given on expert advice.

Tolerance and withdrawal

- Tolerance to benzodiazepines frequently occurs, and there is a prolonged withdrawal syndrome, with:
  - marked anxiety
  - shakiness
  - abdominal cramps
  - perceptual disturbances
  - persecutory delusions
  - seizures.
- They should therefore usually only be prescribed for no more than a couple of weeks. Weaning patients off benzodiazepines to which they have (iatrogenically) become dependent may take months or even years.
- Benzodiazepines inhibit REM sleep and so there is a rebound experienced as increased dreaming when they are stopped.
- Zopiclone and related compounds may also cause dependency and so long-term use should be avoided.

Stimulants

- Methylphenidate is used to treat attention-deficit hyperactivity disorder (ADHD) and, more rarely, narcolepsy.
- Atomoxetine is a newer medication used for treating ADHD (see Chapter 19).
- Side effects of stimulants are:
  - decreased appetite and weight loss
  - anxiety
  - agitation
  - insomnia.

Antidementia drugs

- Drugs currently available to treat the symptoms of Alzheimer's disease (and Lewy body and Parkinson's disease dementia) are:
  - cholinesterase inhibitors (donepezil, rivastigmine and galantamine);
  - memantine (an glutamate receptor antagonist).
- All are given orally. Rivastigmine is also available as a transdermal patch, applied every 24 hours.
- The most common side effects of cholinesterase inhibitors are:
  - gastrointestinal (nausea, diarrhoea, anorexia)
  - dizziness, syncope, bradycardia
  - rash
  - muscle cramps
  - urinary incontinence (and potentially retention).
- The most common side effects of memantine are:
  - constipation
  - hypertension
  - dyspnoea
  - headache
  - dizziness
  - drowsiness.

37 Electroconvulsive Therapy and Other Physical Treatments

Electroconvulsive therapy (ECT)

Mechanism of action

- ECT involves the induction of a modified cerebral seizure. A series of such treatments induces complex effects including:

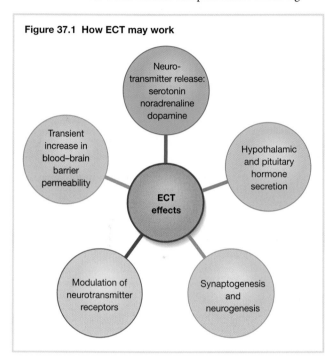

Figure 37.1 How ECT may work

- Neuro-transmitter release: serotonin noradrenaline dopamine
- Transient increase in blood–brain barrier permeability
- Hypothalamic and pituitary hormone secretion
- **ECT effects**
- Modulation of neurotransmitter receptors
- Synaptogenesis and neurogenesis

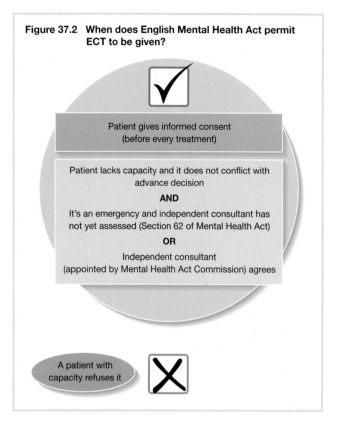

Figure 37.2 When does English Mental Health Act permit ECT to be given?

Patient gives informed consent (before every treatment)

Patient lacks capacity and it does not conflict with advance decision
AND
It's an emergency and independent consultant has not yet assessed (Section 62 of Mental Health Act)
OR
Independent consultant (appointed by Mental Health Act Commission) agrees

A patient with capacity refuses it

Legal aspects

- Figure 37.2 shows when ECT may be given in England and Wales.
- Legal aspects of ECT in other countries are covered in Chapters 40–44.

Indications

- The UK National Institute for Health and Clinical Excellence (NICE) recommends that ECT be used for the treatment of:
  - severe depressive illness (the main indication);
  - a prolonged or severe episode of mania that has not responded to treatment;
  - catatonia;
  - moderate depression that has not responded to multiple drug treatments and psychological treatment.
- ECT should be used to induce fast and short-term improvement of severe symptoms after all other treatment options have failed, or when the situation is thought to be life-threatening (because of high risk of suicide or not eating and drinking).
- Patients with depressive delusions and/or psychomotor retardation are most likely to respond.
- Response rates may be as high as 90%. Speed of response may be faster than that of antidepressants.
- Patients having ECT would nearly always need subsequent treatment for their depression in order to prevent early relapse. This is usually antidepressants and talk therapy.

How is ECT given?

Contraindications

- There are no absolute contraindications to ECT.
- Important relative contraindications are:
  - raised intracranial pressure
  - recent stroke
  - recent myocardial infarction
  - crescendo angina.

Side effects

- Patients have reported that ECT causes cognitive impairment. Therefore cognitive function should be assessed prior to, during and after a course of treatment. Assessment should include:
  - orientation and time to reorientation after each treatment,
  - new learning,
  - retrograde amnesia,
  - subjective memory impairment.
- If there is evidence of significant cognitive impairment at any stage, consider:
  - changing from bilateral to unilateral electrode placement; memory problems are reduced by unilateral electrode placement, though this may be slightly less effective;
  - reducing the stimulus dose;
  - stopping treatment.
- Other side effects include:
  - anaesthetic complications,
  - dysrhythmias due to vagal stimulation,

Psychiatry at a Glance, Sixth Edition. Cornelius Katona, Claudia Cooper, Mary Robertson. © 2016 John Wiley & Sons, Ltd. Published 2016 by John Wiley & Sons, Ltd.
Companion website: www.ataglanceseries.com/psychiatry

- postictal headache,
- confusion,
- retrograde and anterograde amnesia with difficulties in registration and recall that may persist for several weeks.

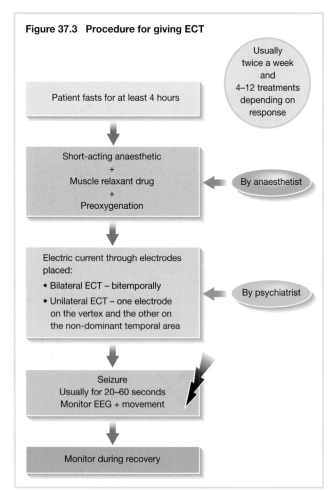

Figure 37.3 Procedure for giving ECT

Patient fasts for at least 4 hours

Usually twice a week and 4–12 treatments depending on response

Short-acting anaesthetic
+
Muscle relaxant drug
+
Preoxygenation

By anaesthetist

Electric current through electrodes placed:
- Bilateral ECT – bitemporally
- Unilateral ECT – one electrode on the vertex and the other on the non-dominant temporal area

By psychiatrist

Seizure
Usually for 20–60 seconds
Monitor EEG + movement

Monitor during recovery

New methods of brain stimulation
Transcranial magnetic stimulation

- The prefrontal cortex is stimulated by the application of a strong magnetic field.
- Treatment usually involves a daily 30-minute session for two to four weeks.
- It does not require a general anaesthetic or analgesia.
- It has shown promise in the treatment of severe depression, although it is still primarily given in a research context.

Vagal nerve stimulation

- This is used in epilepsy and has been employed to treat refractory depression.
- A generator implanted under the skin in the chest area is used to provide electrical stimulation to the nerve.

Deep brain stimulation

- A thin electrode is inserted directly into the brain and currents applied.
- It is used in Parkinson's disease.
- In the USA, it has been used experimentally for obsessive–compulsive disorder (OCD) and Tourette's syndrome.

Neurosurgery for mental disorder

- This is now extremely rare (less than 10 operations a year in the UK). Bilateral anterior capsulotomy or anterior cingulotomy are the only two procedures currently performed.
- Indications are severe treatment-resistant depression and OCD. Success rates of 40–60% are reported.
- There are strict legal constraints to its use in the UK (see Chapters 41–43).

38 Psychiatry in the Community

Most people with mental illness are managed in primary care (if their illness is detected at all). Only those with severe and enduring mental illness are treated by psychiatric services, usually in the community rather than in hospital.

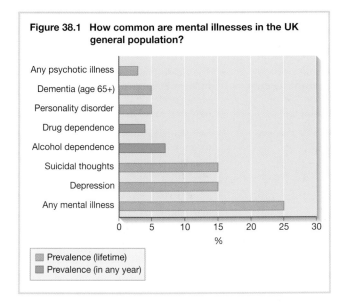

Figure 38.1 How common are mental illnesses in the UK general population?

Psychiatry in primary care

• Psychiatric morbidity doubles the likelihood of primary care consultation, and one in four of these consultations relates to mental health.

• About 30% of significant psychiatric illness is not detected by primary care. Illness is less likely to be detected (and therefore treated) in patients who do not accept that their illness is psychiatric or treatable. Detection may be facilitated in primary care by GPs and other practice staff who:
  • are empathic and understanding;
  • are knowledgeable about mental health;
  • have more time available for consultation;
  • have good communication skills, including appropriate use of eye contact and sensitivity to non-verbal cues;
  • avoid exclusive concentration on the presenting complaint at the expense of any 'hidden agenda'.

• The most common psychiatric illnesses among people attending primary care are depression, anxiety and somatisation disorder (Chapter 27).

• Only about one-eighth of cases detected will be referred to psychiatrists. The decision to refer may reflect the GP's confidence in managing psychiatric illness, the patient's wishes, the accessibility of the psychiatric service and the severity and duration of the illness.

• The challenge of primary care psychiatry is to ensure recognition and optimal care for the submerged iceberg of psychiatric morbidity.

The NHS **Improving Access to Psychological Therapies** (IAPT) programme was introduced to increase the availability of evidence-based psychological treatments for depression and anxiety diagnosed in primary care. Patients are usually offered computer-aided CBT (Chapter 8) or guided self-help, and 'stepped up' to CBT or other evidence-based psychological treatments with a psychological therapist if this does not help. (See http://www.iapt. nhs.uk/services for more information on treatments offered.)

Community care of severe psychiatric illness

• Between 1980 and 1995, large psychiatric hospitals (asylums) closed, and most psychiatric care shifted to the community, supported by fewer, smaller inpatient units. This major change was enabled by:
  • the effectiveness of psychotropic drugs,
  • an ideological commitment to the closure of asylums,
  • the greater cost-effectiveness of community care.

• Since 2000, the number of inpatient beds has declined further as **Crisis Resolution Teams** have been set up to manage severely unwell people at home. Now only those with the most severe illness or highest risk are treated on inpatient wards.

• Most secondary psychiatric care is now delivered by **Community Mental Health Teams** (CMHTs) consisting of psychiatrists, community psychiatric nurses (CPNs), social workers, occupational therapists (OTs) and psychologists.

Specialist psychiatric teams

Many CMHTs are currently undergoing reconfiguration to focus on specific disorders (e.g. psychosis, people with borderline personality disorder). Table 38.1 shows some that are already common in the UK.

Care Programme Approach

• Psychiatric care is managed through the **Care Programme Approach** (CPA) in England, Wales and Scotland (introduced by the 1991 Community Care Act). In Northern Ireland, care plans are reviewed on a regular basis in a similar system.

• CPA meetings take place at least every six months to devise a care plan, documenting:
  • all those involved in a patient's care,
  • the treatment plan,
  • early relapse indicators,
  • a crisis plan should the patient's mental health deteriorate.

• The patient, usually their family and all relevant professionals and services (primarily the health and social services but also housing, GP) are invited.

• Each patient has a nominated **care coordinator** (who may be any member of a CMHT), who arranges the CPA and is responsible for the care plan, seeing the patient regularly (usually monthly). The care coordinator also monitors the patient's mental state and medication adherence, detecting any relapses at an early stage, providing emotional and practical support and promoting the patient's mental well-being (e.g. by avoiding stress, excessive alcohol and drug use).

Psychiatry at a Glance, Sixth Edition. Cornelius Katona, Claudia Cooper, Mary Robertson. © 2016 John Wiley & Sons, Ltd. Published 2016 by John Wiley & Sons, Ltd.
Companion website: www.ataglanceseries.com/psychiatry

Table 38.1 Functions of specialist psychiatric teams

Team	Service they provide	For whom?	What is the aim?
Crisis Resolution Teams (CRTs) (home treatment teams)	Intensive support at home – operate 24 hours a day, and see people about twice a day	People in mental health crises	To prevent admissions and support early discharge
Assertive Outreach Teams (AOTs)	Intensive treatment and support in the community	People who are chronically unwell and have a history of disengaging from services	To provide care to this difficult-to-reach group
Early Intervention in Psychosis Services (EIS)	Intensive treatment for the first two to three years of illness with a focus on promoting return to employment and education	Patients, usually aged 18 to 35, newly diagnosed with psychosis	Promoting recovery in the early stages of psychotic illness, when evidence suggests treatment might be more effective
Community rehabilitation teams	Treatment and support	Adults with especially complex mental health needs	To support this group, who often reside in supported community accommodation and receive inpatient or community rehabilitation for years
Memory services	Diagnosis and management of dementia	People with memory problems	Less than a third of dementia is ever diagnosed; early intervention can improve quality of life and delay institutionalisation

Patient-centred care

- Services aim to provide patient-centred collaborative care, involving patients and their families in treatment decisions, reflecting a shift from previous 'paternalistic' services.
- Many patients find self-help groups beneficial.
- Service users (patients) are increasingly involved in the management of services, training professionals, and advising current patients through **advocacy services**.

Accommodation

- Patients unable to live independently are usually cared for by family or friends (who may themselves need support from services to provide this care).
- There are three main types of supported accommodation:
  - residential/nursing care homes,
  - supported housing (individual or shared accommodation with staff on-site),
  - floating outreach (support of a specified number of hours per week not tied to accommodation).
- These services are usually run by social services, voluntary and independent sector organisations.
- The amount of professional support varies from 24-hour nursed care (residential/nursing homes) to mental health workers visiting two or three times per week (floating outreach services).
- Most aim to provide rehabilitation so that people can return to independent living or less supported settings.

- The assessment of people's ability to care for themselves (e.g. personal hygiene, shopping, budgeting, cooking, cleaning) and the nature of their illness is important in deciding what level of support they will need to live successfully in the community and avoid relapse and return to hospital.

Daytime activity

- Employment is important for mental health, as it brings:
  - income
  - purpose
  - daytime structure
  - social networks.
- Barriers to accessing employment are anxiety, a lack of motivation, concerns about losing state benefits and discrimination.
- Discrimination is an important barrier, even though the **Disability Discrimination Act 1995** prohibits employers from treating people with chronic (including mental) illness differently.
- Most services now focus on supporting people with mental health problems to obtain employment, attend college courses or train for work.
- **Support, Time and Recovery (STaR)** workers help service users to access a range of daytime activities. Many STaR workers are ex-service users and provide expertise through their experience of mental health problems to give service users peer support as well as helping them access daytime activities.

39 Forensic Psychiatry

Forensic psychiatry concerns the legal aspects of mental disorders. The forensic psychiatrist is primarily concerned with the assessment, treatment and rehabilitation of mentally disordered offenders. Legal competence is discussed in Chapter 40.

Crime and mental disorder

- Most mentally ill people are never dangerous. They are far more likely to be victims than perpetrators of crime.
- People with mental illness commit proportionately fewer violent crimes than those without such illness.
- Mental disorder may increase the likelihood of arrest because of decreased ability to avoid detection or to negotiate an alternative outcome.

Schizophrenia

- There is an association with violent crime, which is mostly accounted for by a higher frequency of substance misuse in people with schizophrenia than in the general population.

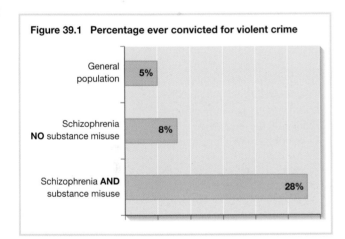

Figure 39.1 Percentage ever convicted for violent crime

General population	5%
Schizophrenia **NO** substance misuse	8%
Schizophrenia **AND** substance misuse	28%

- Up to 10% of homicide offenders may have schizophrenia, but, as violent crime is rare, the annual risk that a person with schizophrenia will commit a homicide is low (about 1 in 10 000).
- The rate of homicide in 15 times higher in psychosis if the illness is untreated.
- Arson is much more commonly perpetrated by people with schizophrenia than by members of the general population.

Affective disorder

- Severe **depression** can lead to hopelessness and a view that death is the only solution.
- Depression-related homicide is rare, usually domestic (often infanticide), in response to delusions (e.g. believing that the victim is fatally ill and suffering) and often followed by suicide.
- Offences linked to **mania** may reflect financial irresponsibility (fraud, defaulted debt) or impulsivity (shoplifting, occasionally violence).

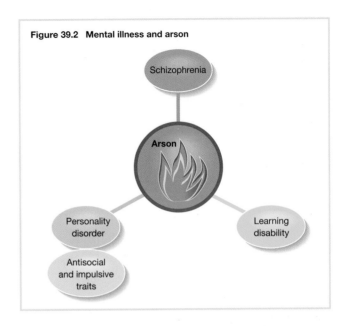

Figure 39.2 Mental illness and arson

- Schizophrenia
- Arson
- Personality disorder
- Learning disability
- Antisocial and impulsive traits

Alcohol and substance misuse

- These are strongly associated with violent crime and driving offences.
- Theft, robbery and shoplifting may be motivated by a lack of funds to buy illicit drugs.
- Alcohol is often implicated in **morbid or pathological jealousy** (see Chapter 18), which may culminate in spousal homicide.

Cognitive disorders

- **Dementia** is occasionally associated with shoplifting (forgetting to pay) and sexual offences (usually reflecting frontal disinhibition).
- Subjects with **learning disability** (see Chapter 24) may commit sexual offences or arson.

Personality disorders

- There is a strong association between crime and **antisocial personality disorder,** although this assertion is somewhat circular since offending may be integral to the diagnosis.
- Individuals with severe emotionally unstable, impulsive, paranoid and histrionic personality traits are more likely than others to offend.
- Shoplifting has been associated with poor impulse control (e.g. in antisocial personality disorder).

Managing violence (see also Chapter 4)
Assessing risk of violence

- This is important when assessing for compulsory detention, transferring patients between different levels of security and planning aftercare.
- Pay attention to the forensic history and distinguish:
  - crimes against property and violence against the person,

Psychiatry at a Glance, Sixth Edition. Cornelius Katona, Claudia Cooper, Mary Robertson. © 2016 John Wiley & Sons, Ltd. Published 2016 by John Wiley & Sons, Ltd.
Companion website: www.ataglanceseries.com/psychiatry

- crimes occurring during periods of illness and during remissions,
- precursors to past violence and their risk of recurrence.

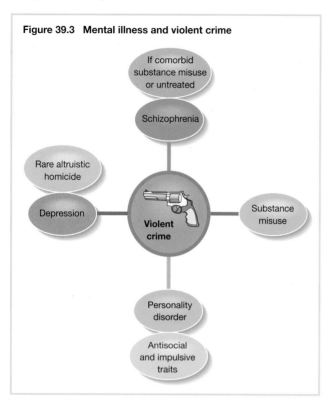

Figure 39.3   Mental illness and violent crime

- While a history of violence is a strong predictor of risk subsequently, a first episode of violence can occur in the context of severe stress or a psychotic disorder.
- Risk may have to be managed by compulsory detention, sometimes long term. Resource issues should not be allowed to cloud judgements about the management of violence.

Managing mental illness in the criminal justice system

- Psychiatric illnesses, particularly psychoses and drug- or alcohol-related disorders, are overrepresented in prisoners. This partly reflects a group of urban, homeless, psychiatrically ill, multiple reoffenders (see Chapter 24 for more on mental health of prisoners).
- Half to two-thirds of prisoners have a personality disorder.
- Most prisoners with mental illness are managed by prison-based primary and mental health services.
- The forensic sections of the Mental Health Act are used where prisoners are judged to require transfer to psychiatric hospital (Chapters 41–44).

Managing offenders and potentially violent patients in the psychiatric services

- **Court diversion schemes** seek to ensure that mentally ill people who are brought before the courts obtain appropriate care from health and social services.
- Psychiatric inpatients judged to be too high a risk for general psychiatric or psychiatric intensive care units (PICUs) are managed in:
    - **medium (or regional) secure units**, or (where the risk is greatest)
    - **high secure hospitals** (Broadmoor, Ashworth, Rampton and Carstairs in the UK).
- Some UK prisons (and Broadmoor and Rampton high secure hospitals) have specialist units for the treatment of people with **dangerous severe personality disorders**. These are for prisoners who present a serious risk to others as a result of a personality disorder.

Prostitution

- Prostitution is not in itself illegal, but it is illegal to loiter or solicit sex on the street.
- Women who work as prostitutes are at high risk of mental illness.

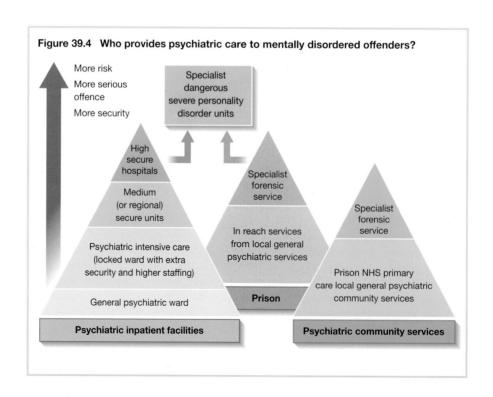

Figure 39.4   Who provides psychiatric care to mentally disordered offenders?

40 Mental Capacity

- In health and social care, as in other areas of life, people are generally presumed to have capacity to make their own decisions unless there is reason to believe they do not. Capacity should be assessed carefully so that patients who are able to make their own decisions are not denied their right to do so, and those without capacity receive good health and social care.
- In some countries, a legal framework governs the process by which carers and professionals make welfare, health care and financial decisions on behalf of people who lack capacity. These laws seek to protect vulnerable people from harm, neglect and exploitation. In other countries there is no specific legislation, and decisions are made under common law.

Assessing capacity

- A person may lack capacity to make a decision as a result of any cause that impairs reasoning ability, be it temporary or permanent (e.g. dementia, intellectual disability, acute confusional state).
- A person lacks capacity to make a decision if he or she is unable to:
  - understand information relevant to the decision;
  - retain, use and weigh that information to come to a decision;
  - communicate that decision (by talking, sign language or other means).
- If a lack of capacity is likely to be temporary, it may be possible to delay the decision until the person can make it themselves.
- People should always be helped to make decisions for themselves where they have the capacity to do so, and to give their views where possible if they do not.
- Assessment of capacity should be repeated because a person's capacity to make a decision can change with time.

The Mental Capacity Act (England and Wales)

Figure 40.1 What does the Mental Capacity Act (2005) (England and Wales) do?

Gives any adult with capacity the right to make
- Advance decision(s)
- Lasting power of attorney

AND

Says how to decide if someone has capacity

AND

For any adult without capacity it tells professionals to
- Act in their best interests
- Consult family/friends about decisions
- Appoint IMCA for important decisions
- Apply Deprivation of Liberty Safeguards (DoLS) to anyone deprived of liberty

---

If a person lacks capacity, professionals must make decisions in their best interests.
- Professionals have a duty to consult carers and family. If the person has no one to speak for them, an independent mental capacity advocate (IMCA) is appointed to represent their wishes on important issues of welfare and health.

Lasting Power of Attorney (LPA)

- This allows a person with capacity to appoint an attorney to make these decisions on their behalf if they lose capacity.
- The attorney (usually a relative or friend) can be directed by the person appointing them to make decisions about their property and financial affairs and their personal welfare, which includes health care and where they live.

Advance decisions

- Anyone with capacity can make an advance decision (also sometimes called an 'advance directive') about treatment they do not want to receive in the future if they lose capacity to make treatment decisions.
- This can include life-saving treatment so long as this is specified by the person making the advance decision.
- Advance decisions permit a person to refuse treatment but not to demand it.

Deprivation of liberty safeguards (DoLS)

- These apply to people in hospitals and care homes who:
  - are deprived of their liberty (not allowed to come and go as they please),
  - lack capacity to consent to the confinement,
  - are not sectioned under the Mental Health Act (MHA).
- When a hospital or care home identifies that a person who lacks capacity is being, or risks being, deprived of their liberty, they must apply for an authorisation of deprivation of liberty. Authorisation is only granted if two assessors agree that:
  - the person is aged 18 or over;
  - it would not conflict with a valid decision by a donee of Lasting Power of Attorney, a deputy appointed by the Court of Protection, or an advance decision;
  - the person lacks capacity to decide whether to be admitted to, or remain in, the hospital or care home;
  - the person is suffering from a mental disorder;
  - the person is not detained under the MHA;
  - the application is not to enable mental health treatment in hospital of someone who objects to being in hospital or to the treatment (in which case the MHA should be considered);
  - it is in the person's best interests, and necessary and proportionate to prevent harm to them.
- Authorisations must be renewed at least annually.
- The patient (or their representative) may appeal; the Court of Protection has the powers to terminate the order or vary the conditions.

Psychiatry at a Glance, Sixth Edition. Cornelius Katona, Claudia Cooper, Mary Robertson. © 2016 John Wiley & Sons, Ltd. Published 2016 by John Wiley & Sons, Ltd.
Companion website: www.ataglanceseries.com/psychiatry

Legal competence

Most mentally ill people retain responsibility for their actions and the capacity to manage their affairs. However, careful assessment of capacity is crucial to the criminal justice system.

Fitness to plead

- This is for a jury to decide.
- It refers to a defendant's competence to mount a defence against charges.

The Adults with Incapacity (Scotland) Act 2000

This sets out similar legislation for appointing a Power of Attorney to look after one's property and financial affairs and/or to make specified decisions about personal welfare, including medical treatment. The Act gives sheriffs power to grant guardianship orders dealing with 'all aspects' of the personal welfare of an adult. The guardian can arrange for the adult's return to the place where he or she is required to live and can obtain a court order requiring the adult to comply with the guardian's decisions. In practice these powers are used to detain people without capacity, although unlike the English and Welsh law, deprivation of liberty is not specifically mentioned in the act.

The Enduring Powers of Attorney (Northern Ireland) Order 1987

This allows for the appointment of an attorney to make decisions regarding financial and property matters only (Enduring Power of Attorney). There is no specific legislation governing management of health and welfare of people without capacity in Northern Ireland, although the planned Mental Capacity (Health, Welfare and Finance) Bill (see Chapter 43) will address this.

- People are deemed fit to plead if they have the capacity to:
  - understand the charge
  - distinguish between guilty and not guilty pleas
  - instruct lawyers
  - follow court evidence
  - challenge jurors.
- If a person is found unfit to plead, a trial of the facts may still take place, and the defendant would be acquitted if the facts were not established. If the facts are proven, there may be flexibility in the sentence imposed.

Mens rea

- For guilt (of most crimes) to be established, it is necessary to demonstrate that the defendant was 'criminally responsible', possessing the *mens rea* (guilty mind) to commit the offence.
- *Mens rea* may be absent by virtue of:
  - **age** – children under 10 years cannot be criminally responsible, and for those aged 10–14 years the prosecution must prove *mens rea*;
  - **lack of criminal intent** (e.g. accidents);

- **automatism** – this refers to dissociation between mind and action (e.g. epilepsy, sleepwalking, concussion);

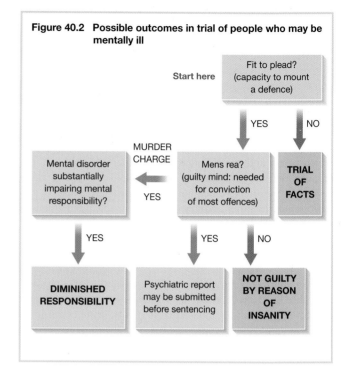

Figure 40.2 Possible outcomes in trial of people who may be mentally ill

- **mental disorder** – this is rarely invoked to deny *mens rea*; it must be established that the defendant was mentally ill at the time of the offence, resulting in a 'defect of reason or disease of the mind', and that consequently he/she could not tell what he/she was doing or know that it was wrong. If successful, the verdict is '**not guilty by reason of insanity**'. This theoretically allows some flexibility of sentence, although it usually results in hospital detention.

Diminished responsibility

- In murder, conviction may be modified to manslaughter on grounds of **diminished responsibility** on the basis of specific 'abnormality of mind' substantially impairing mental responsibility. This is defined as 'arising from a condition of arrested or retarded development of mind or any inherent causes or induced by disease or injury'.

Testamentary capacity

- Testamentary capacity (capacity/competence to make a will) must be present for a will to be valid.
- It requires a person to:
  - understand the act of making a will,
  - appreciate the extent of his/her property and assets,
  - be aware of who might have a reasonable claim on their estate.
- If the person is mentally ill, testamentary capacity implies that his/her judgement should not be clouded regarding the will itself. Delusions or hallucinations only impair testamentary capacity where they are directly relevant to the will (e.g. delusions of poverty).

Mental Health Legislation in England and Wales

Table 41.1 Summary of main civil (not forensic) sections

MHA section	Purpose	Recommendation(s)	Applicant	Duration
2	Assessment	2 doctors	AMHP or nearest relative (NR)	28 days
3	Treatment	2 doctors	AMHP or NR	6 months
Community Treatment Order	Treatment in community of patient previously detained on Section 3 or 37		Responsible clinician (agreed with AMHP)	6 months
4	Urgent assessment from community (no time to arrange Section 2)	1 doctor (AC)	AMHP or NR	72 hours
5(2)	Urgent detention of inpatient	1 doctor		72 hours
5(4)	Urgent detention of psychiatric inpatient in absence of doctor	Registered mental nurse		6 hours
135	Removal from home to place of safety	Police officer		72 hours
136	Removal from public place to place of safety	Police officer		72 hours

- The Mental Health Act (MHA) 1983 (amended by the MHA 2007) is concerned with the care and treatment of patients compulsorily detained in hospital and those under community treatment orders.
- It is supervised by the Mental Health Act Commission (MHAC).

Sectioning (compulsory admission)

- Compulsory admission ('sectioning') requires that:
  - a patient is judged to have a mental disorder sufficiently severe to need detention in hospital in the interests of his/her own health/safety, or for the protection of others;
  - for patients to be detained under the longer lasting sections (e.g. Sections 3, 37) *appropriate medical treatment must be available to them*;
  - people cannot be detained because of learning disability alone unless it is associated with abnormally aggressive or seriously irresponsible conduct.

Mental disorder is defined as any disorder or disability of the mind. It includes mental illness, personality disorder, learning disability and disorders of sexual preference (e.g. paedophilia), but NOT dependence on alcohol or drugs.

How 'sectioning' is carried out

- Most hospital detentions are under Sections 2 or 3:
  - *Section 2*: admission for assessment (or assessment followed by treatment), lasts up to 28 days.
  - *Section 3*: admission for treatment, lasts up to six months (renewable).
- Application for these sections is made by an **Approved Mental Health Professional (AMHP)**. AMHPs may be social workers, nurses, psychologists or occupational therapists (not doctors). Rarely, the nearest relative may make the application.
- Application is made on the recommendations of two medical practitioners, one of whom should be 'approved' under Section 12 (for which specialist experience and completion of a training course is required) and one of whom should have 'previous knowledge/acquaintance' of/with the patient (e.g. the patient's GP). Doctors

with 'previous knowledge/acquaintance' may also complete the recommendations even if they are not Section 12 approved.
- For Section 3, the AMHP has a duty to consult the nearest relative if possible, and, if they object, the section cannot proceed unless the **responsible clinician** (RC: person responsible for care under section, generally consultant psychiatrist) takes legal action to displace the nearest relative.
- MHA assessments are convened by the AMHP, usually at the patient's home or in hospital. Two ACs and the AMHP assess the patient; if they decide that the patient should be in hospital and the patient refuses informal admission, they arrange admission under section.
- Police may attend assessments if there are concerns that the patient will be violent or physically resist coming to hospital if detained.
- Where a patient lacks capacity to agree to an informal admission (e.g. because of dementia), the patient may still be admitted informally so long as she/he appears to assent and does not object. Such admission would be subject to the provisions of **Deprivation of Liberty Safeguards (DoLS)** (see Chapter 40).

Emergency sections

These last for up to 72 hours, except Section 5(4) which lasts six hours:
- *Section 4* is used when admission (otherwise fulfilling Section 2 requirements) is more urgent than Section 2 procedures would allow.
- *Section 136* empowers a police officer who finds a person in a public place appearing to suffer from a mental disorder to remove him/her to a 'place of safety' for assessment.
- *Section 135* empowers a police officer or other authorised person acting on a magistrate's warrant to enter premises and remove to a place of safety a person who is believed to be suffering from a mental disorder.
- *Section 5(2)*, for patients already in hospital (any ward but not A&E), is on the recommendation of the RC or his/her nominated deputy. Patients placed on Section 5(2) must subsequently be assessed for Sections 2 or 3 or discharged from Section 5(2) to become an informal patient.

Psychiatry at a Glance, Sixth Edition. Cornelius Katona, Claudia Cooper, Mary Robertson. © 2016 John Wiley & Sons, Ltd. Published 2016 by John Wiley & Sons, Ltd.
Companion website: www.ataglanceseries.com/psychiatry

Section 5(4) allows urgent detention for <6 hours of a patient already receiving treatment for mental disorder in hospital, on the recommendation of a registered mental nurse when a doctor is not able to attend immediately.

Community treatment

- **Community Treatment Order (CTO)**: patients may be placed on a CTO following detention in hospital under Sections 3 or 37, by application of the RC with agreement of the AMHP. CTOs require that patients make themselves available for medical examination. Patients may be recalled to hospital if they require treatment on grounds of their health or safety that can only be given in hospital; refuse to make themselves available for examination by the RC or do not comply with conditions of the CTO. Once recalled they may be detained for up to 72 hours for assessment. During that time, the RC must either revoke the CTO (the patient returns to being detained under Sections 3 or 37) or release the patient. Alternatively the patient may agree to an informal admission.
- **Guardianship (Sections 7 and 8)**: a guardian (usually an AMHP), nominated by the local authority, is empowered to ensure that an individual resides at a specified place, attends specified places and times for treatment, education, training or occupation and allows specified people (e.g. AMHPs, doctors) access to their residence.

Leave and discharge from section

- **Section 17** requires that patients on Sections 2 or 3 can only have leave subject to the RC's specific instructions.
- Patients may be discharged from a section before it expires by:
  - the *RC*;
  - a *Mental Health Review Tribunal (MHRT)*, to whom patients may appeal, within 14 days for Section 2 or at any time within the first six months and once during each subsequent period of renewal for Section 3 (MHRTs consist of a lawyer (president), psychiatrist and a lay member (for Section 41 patients the president is a judge or Queen's Counsel)); patients may be granted legal aid and obtain an independent medical opinion;
  - the *Mental Health Act managers* (community members who act as non-executive directors of a hospital) for discharge, if patients appeal to them;
  - the *nearest relative*, although they must give 72 hours' notice and can be barred in some circumstances by the RC.

Forensic sections

- Here are the main sections of the MHA relating to those charged with or convicted of crimes.

Table 41.2 Summary of main forensic sections

Section	What does it do?	Recommendation(s)	Who applies?	Length
35	Remands an accused person to hospital for a report	1 doctor	Crown or Magistrates' Court	28 days
36	Remands an accused person to hospital for treatment appropriate medical treatment must be available	2 doctors (1 approved)	Crown Court	28 days
37	Orders a hospital admission or guardianship of a person convicted of an imprisonable offence (except murder)	2 doctors	Crown or Magistrates' Court	6 months
38	Sends convicted person to hospital for treatment prior to sentencing	2 doctors	Crown or Magistrates' Court	28 days
41	Applies restriction that patient on another hospital section may not be given leave, transferred or discharged, without the Home Secretary's consent	1 doctor	Crown Court	Duration of other section
47	Transfers sentenced prisoner to hospital for treatment	2 doctors	Home office	6 months

Treatment without consent

- Except in emergencies, patients detained under the emergency sections (e.g. 5(2), 135, 136, 4) may not be treated without their consent.

- Here are the sections that allow treatment without consent and what they say:

Table 41.3 Provisions for treatment without consent

Section	Type of treatment	What it says
2 and 3 (and equivalent forensic sections)	Medication for first three months	May be given without consent
58	Medication on sections 2 and 3 after three months	Patient must consent (and be attested competent to do so by the **RC**)
	ECT at any time	**OR** an independent **Second Opinion Approved Doctor (SOAD)** nominated by the MHAC must:
		interview the patient
		discuss the treatment with the RC and two other professionals involved in the patient's treatment
		agree the treatment is necessary
		ECT cannot be given to patients with capacity without their consent
57	Psychosurgery	Needs both consent and a second opinion
	Surgical hormone implants	
62	Life-saving treatment	Exempt from Sections 57 and 58

Mental Health Legislation in Scotland

- **The Mental Health (Care and Treatment) (Scotland) Act 2003** concerns the compulsory treatment of people with mental disorders living in Scotland. It amends the Criminal Procedure (Scotland) Act 1995 regarding the treatment of mentally disordered offenders.
- The Mental Welfare Commission is an independent body that monitors the operation of the Act and promotes best practice. It appoints designated medical practitioners when circumstances require a second medical opinion on compulsory treatment.
- The 2003 Act gives people with a mental disorder a right to independent **advocacy**. Additionally, any adult can appoint a **named person** (if this is agreed in writing and witnessed) who has a right to be consulted and to appeal against the detention of the person they support.
- The Act also allows people to make **advance statements** about how they would wish to be treated if they became unable to express their views as a result of becoming mentally unwell. The Mental Health Tribunal and doctors treating the person must take notice of an advance statement and inform the patient, the patient's named person and the Mental Welfare Commission in writing of the reasons if they do not follow it.

Compulsory orders

- To be detained:
  - a person must be suffering from a mental disorder (mental illness (including dementia), personality disorder or learning disability) that:
    - significantly impairs their decision making with respect to medical treatment of the disorder, and
    - would put their health, safety or welfare, or the safety of another, at significant risk if they were not detained.
  - detention must be deemed necessary.
- Significantly impaired decision-making ability is not the same as 'incapacity' under the Adults with Incapacity (Scotland) Act 2000 (see Chapter 40), but it is a related concept. It refers to the specific capacity of an individual to make decisions about medical treatment for mental disorder, whereas the Adults with Incapacity (Scotland) Act 2000 covers a range of different capacities.

Here are the main compulsory orders.
- a **Mental Health Officer (MHO)** (a social worker with additional training),
- an **Approved Medical Practitioner (AMP)** (a doctor with mental health expertise, usually a psychiatrist).

Compulsory Treatment Orders

- Compulsory Treatment Orders (CTOs) require that medical treatment is available that may prevent deterioration, or help treat any symptoms or effects of the mental disorder, and without which there would be a significant risk to the person or others. Medical treatment may include nursing care, psychological intervention, education and training in living skills. It lasts up to six months initially, can be extended for a further six months, and subsequently for 12 months at a time. It may be based in hospital or the community. A community order may require the patient to receive medical treatment (but not by force), live at a certain address and attend certain services for treatment.
- The decision on whether to grant a CTO is made by the Mental Health Tribunal. Tribunals have three panel members: a lawyer, a doctor with experience in mental health and a third person with other skills and experience. An MHO makes an application to the Tribunal, including two medical recommendations and a proposed care plan. Patients are given the opportunity to express their views at the Tribunal, if they wish to.
- If the Tribunal needs further information before making a final decision, or the patient or their solicitor needs more time to prepare their case, the Tribunal may make an **interim (temporary) CTO** (<28 days), which can be renewed once only.

How orders are ended

- If the person no longer fulfils the criteria, short-term detention and CTOs can be cancelled by:
  - the Responsible Medical Officer (a medical practitioner, usually a consultant psychiatrist and AMP),
  - the Mental Welfare Commission, or
  - the Mental Health Review Tribunal. The patient or their named person has the right to appeal against decisions made by the Tribunal.

Table 42.1 The main compulsory orders

MHA order	Purpose	Location	Requirements	Maximum duration
Emergency detention	Detention for urgent assessment if arranging short-term detention order would involve undesirable delay	Hospital	Certification by any fully registered doctor Agreement of an MHO if possible	72 hours
Short-term detention	Assessment or treatment	Hospital	Recommendation by an AMP Agreement of an MHO	28 days
Compulsory Treatment Order	Treatment	Hospital or community	Recommendation by two AMPs Application by MHO Decision by Mental Health Review Tribunal	6 months

Psychiatry at a Glance, Sixth Edition. Cornelius Katona, Claudia Cooper, Mary Robertson. © 2016 John Wiley & Sons, Ltd. Published 2016 by John Wiley & Sons, Ltd.
Companion website: www.ataglanceseries.com/psychiatry

Other short-term holding powers

- **Nurses' holding power** – an appropriately qualified nurse can hold a hospital patient who has been receiving treatment on a voluntary basis for up to two hours to allow a doctor to assess the patient. This can be extended by another one hour once the doctor arrives.
- **Removal to place of safety** – the police can take a person from a public place to a place of safety for <24 hours for assessment if the person appears to have a mental disorder and to be in need of care and treatment.

Mental health law relating to prisoners

- The court can make assessment and treatment orders at any stage of the criminal justice process prior to sentencing. Here are the main orders:
- The court may detain a person who has been acquitted of an offence but who may require admission to hospital for treatment of a mental disorder in a place of safety for <6 hours so a medical examination can be carried out.

Medical treatment

- Urgent treatment that is not associated with significant risks or irreversible consequences may be given without consent to save a patient's life, to alleviate serious suffering on the part of the patient or to prevent violent or dangerous behaviour. Where a detained patient does not or cannot consent to drug treatment, it must be authorised by an independent medical practitioner to continue beyond two months.
- Electroconvulsive therapy (ECT) may only be given to a patient if he or she can and does consent, or is incapable of consenting and the treatment is authorised by an independent medical practitioner. ECT cannot be given to a patient who has capacity and refuses the treatment, even in an emergency.
- Neurosurgery for mental disorder can only be carried out after an independent medical practitioner gives an opinion that it will be beneficial to the patient, and two lay people appointed by the Commission have certified that the person consents, or does not object if they are incapable of giving consent. Where the person is incapable of consenting, the Court of Session must also give approval.

Table 42.2 The main assessment and treatment orders

MHA order	Purpose	Location	Requirements	Maximum duration
Assessment	Assessment	Hospital	Made by court Evidence from one doctor	28 days
Interim compulsion	Longer period of assessment	Hospital	Made by court Evidence from two doctors (one an AMP)	1 year (renewal every 12 weeks)
Treatment	Treatment	Hospital	Made by court Evidence from two doctors (one an AMP)	Until end of remand period or sentence
Compulsion	Similar to a CTO (see above), except the requirement for significantly impaired decision-making ability with regard to treatment does not apply	Hospital	Made by court Evidence from two doctors (one an AMP) Report from the designated MHO	6 months
Restriction	Any change in the legal status of the patient must be referred to Scottish Ministers and the Tribunal	Hospital		Added to compulsion order
Transfer for treatment directions	Transfer of prisoners to hospital for mental health treatment	Hospital	Made by Scottish ministers Evidence from two doctors (one an AMP)	Until sentence expires

Mental Health Legislation in Northern Ireland

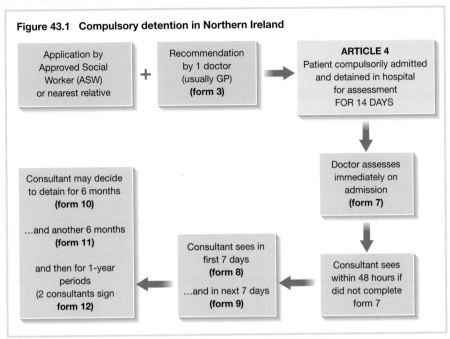

Figure 43.1 Compulsory detention in Northern Ireland

- *The 1986 Mental Health (Northern Ireland) Order* makes provision for the detention, guardianship, care and treatment of patients. Its use is monitored by the Mental Health Commission of Northern Ireland.
- The Mental Capacity (Health, Welfare and Finance) Bill, which it is hoped will be enacted in 2015 will replace the 1986 Mental Health Order. It will reform mental health legislation and develop new capacity legislation. At the time of writing, the 1986 Mental Health (Northern Ireland) Order remains in force.

Criteria for detention

- The definition of mental disorder comprises mental illness, mental handicap, severe mental handicap and severe mental impairment. Mental illness is defined as a 'state of mind which affects a person's thinking, perceiving, emotion or judgement to the extent that he requires care or medical treatment in his own interests or the interests of other persons'. The order cannot be used for the compulsory treatment of addictions, personality disorders (unlike the legislation in England, Wales or Scotland) or sexual deviancy, unless the above criteria are also met.
- People may be detained only if:
  - they are suffering from a mental disorder of a nature or degree that warrants detention in hospital for assessment (or for assessment followed by medical treatment),
  - failure to detain the patient would create a substantial likelihood of serious physical harm to the patient or to others.
- Criteria for likelihood of serious physical harm are that the patient has inflicted, or threatened or attempted to inflict, serious physical harm on themselves; the patient's judgement is so affected that they are, or would soon be, unable to protect themselves against serious physical harm, and that reasonable

provision for their protection is not available in the community; or that other persons have reasonable fear they may suffer serious physical harm owing to violent or other behaviour of the person.

Compulsory admission to hospital

- *Article 4* permits a patient to be compulsorily admitted and detained in hospital for assessment on the application of the nearest relative or an approved social worker (ASW).
- This application must be supported by the recommendation of one doctor (who completes a Form 3) and the doctor and ASW must have seen the patient in the two days preceding the application.
- The doctor should (if possible) know the patient and (except in cases of urgent necessity) not be on the staff of the receiving hospital. In practice, the doctor is usually the patient's GP.
- All detained patients are initially admitted for a period of assessment of up to 14 days.
- A doctor must assess the patient immediately after admission to hospital (and complete a Form 7).
- If the admitting doctor is not a consultant, the patient must be seen by a consultant within 48 hours of admission.
- If the patient is further detained, he or she will be seen again by a consultant within the first and second seven-day periods of the admission (the consultant will complete a Form 8 and a Form 9 for these respective time periods).
- The consultant may then complete a Form 10, which allows detention for treatment (six months in the first instance). This may be extended for a second six-month period (Form 11), and thereafter for periods of one year (for which a Form 12 must be signed by two consultants).

Psychiatry at a Glance, Sixth Edition. Cornelius Katona, Claudia Cooper, Mary Robertson. © 2016 John Wiley & Sons, Ltd. Published 2016 by John Wiley & Sons, Ltd.
Companion website: www.ataglanceseries.com/psychiatry

Police powers

- A police officer may remove from a public place an individual who appears to be suffering from a mental disorder and in need of immediate care and control and take the person to a place of safety (usually a police station), where he or she must be seen by a doctor and ASW.
- If the person is not in a public place and access to the property is denied, a warrant to enter the premises may be obtained (Article 129) by an ASW, another officer of the Health and Social Services Trust or a police officer from a Justice of the Peace.
- If the police officer has to enter the premises, by force or otherwise, he or she must be accompanied by a medical practitioner (usually a GP) who will administer medical treatment if required. The person may then be transferred to a place of safety.

Informal hospital patients

- A patient who has been admitted informally and subsequently wants to leave or refuse treatment may be detained if appropriate by completion of a Form 5 or 5a (for psychiatric and general hospital patients respectively), usually by a junior doctor.
- The patient's own GP (or another practitioner who has previous knowledge of the patient) must then attend the hospital to complete a medical recommendation (Form 3), and an ASW or nearest relative must make an application, after which matters proceed as for other detained patients.
- A doctor on the staff of the hospital in which it is intended that the assessment should be carried out cannot give the recommendation except in a case of urgent necessity.

Guardianship

- A guardianship order may require the patient to:
  - reside at a certain place;
  - attend at specified places and times for the purpose of medical treatment, occupation, education or training;
  - allow any specified doctor, ASW or other person access to their residence.
- The order lasts for six months initially, and may then be renewed for a further six months and yearly thereafter.
- Persons aged 16 or over may be subject to a guardianship order if they are found to be suffering from mental illness or severe mental handicap and it is deemed necessary in the interests of their welfare.
- The application may be made by an ASW or a patient's nearest relative, who must have personally seen the patient within 14 days of the application, and be supported by two medical recommendations.
- The ASW should consult the nearest relative if possible. If the nearest relative objects, involvement of a second ASW is required.
- The nominated guardian is normally a social worker.

Patients involved in criminal proceedings

- Courts may remand an unsentenced prisoner to hospital for two weeks for the preparation of reports (Article 42) or for treatment (Article 43).
- A remand under Article 42 can be made on the basis of one medical opinion – the oral evidence of a Part II-approved doctor (in practice, a consultant). Article 42 does not allow treatment without the patient's consent, or granting of temporary leave from the hospital.
- The court may make a hospital or guardianship order or hospital order with restriction when sentencing a prisoner (Article 44) on receipt of evidence from two medical practitioners, one of whom must be Part II-approved and give oral evidence. An interim hospital order allows admission to hospital before the court makes a hospital order.
- A person serving a sentence of imprisonment may be transferred to hospital for treatment after two written reports have been provided to the Secretary of State (Article 53). Article 53 requires 'that the person is suffering from mental illness or severe mental impairment'.

Appeal

- The Mental Health Review Tribunal hears appeals against detention in hospital or guardianship orders. It consists of a legal member who is the president, a medical member and a lay member.
- Referral to the Tribunal may be by the patient or nearest relative and the hospital trust must refer any patient who has been detained for two years without a tribunal hearing.
- Under the 1986 Order, the patient needed to prove that he or she should be released. This was found to be incompatible with the European Convention on Human Rights. The Mental Health (Amendment) (Northern Ireland) Order 2004 has therefore amended the 1986 Order to shift the burden of proof to the health and social services trust to demonstrate that a patient should *not* be discharged.

Consent to treatment

- This legislation is similar to the 1983 Mental Health Act (England and Wales) provision (Chapter 41).
- *Article 63* states that patients may not receive neurosurgery for mental disorder unless they consent and the treatment is recommended in a second opinion from an independent doctor. These safeguards apply to both detained patients and voluntary patients.
- *Article 64* covers other serious forms of treatment and requires either the patient's consent or a second medical opinion (e.g. for electroconvulsive therapy (ECT)). These requirements apply only to detained patients.
- *Article 68* deals with cases requiring urgent treatment necessary for certain specified emergencies (e.g. ECT) which may be given without the patient's consent or a second medical opinion.

44 Mental Health Legislation in Australia and New Zealand

Each Australian state and territory as well as New Zealand has its own Mental Health Act (MHA), upholding the rights and interests of people with mental illness. Definitions of mental illness, disorder and distress vary between jurisdictions but each act sets a standard that must be met for detention and considers risk to self or others, and the need to provide the least restrictive form of care.

Requirements for detention

Table 44.1 lists the sections relevant to the assessment and detention of a person under the MHA, in each of the Australian States and Territories and in New Zealand.

A medical practitioner (MP)'s ability to provide treatment without consent

In each jurisdiction there is statutory provision for authorised MPs or other persons or bodies (e.g. Guardianship Board (TAS), responsible clinician (NZ)) to give treatment to involuntary patients, usually in approved mental health facilities. The treatment may be for mental illness or disorder (all jurisdictions) and, in some jurisdictions (e.g. NSW, SA), for any other illness.

Community treatment orders (CTOs) and the role of medical practitioners

Community treatment or community care orders impose varying requirements on mental health patients to accept medication and therapy, counselling, management, rehabilitation and other services while living in the community.

New South Wales (NSW): A CTO may be made by the Mental Health Review Tribunal (MHRT) or a magistrate and is valid for up to one year. The director of community treatment (who may be an MP) may initiate breach proceedings.

South Australia (SA): A Level 1 CTO may be made by an MP if the patient meets the requirements of the MHA. It is valid for 28 days if made by a psychiatrist or an authorised MP. An application for a Level 2 CTO may be made by an MP to the Guardianship Tribunal and is valid for up to one year.

Table 44.1 Detention under the Mental Health Act

Jurisdiction	Key sections	Procedures
NSW **Mental Health Act 2007**	General restrictions on detention (ss12–13) Mental illness (s14) Mental disorder (s15)	Detained in a declared mental health facility on the certificate of a medical practitioner (MP)
QLD **Mental Health Act 2000**	Assessment criteria (s13) Mental illness (s12)	Recommendation made by a MP who has examined the person in the last 3 days (in force for 7 days)
SA **Mental Health Act 2009**	Orders for admission and detention (s12) Mental illness (s3)	A MP may make an order (3 days duration) for detention of a person
WA **Mental Health Act 1996**	Involuntary patients (s26) Mental illness (s4)	A MP in specific circumstances can refer a person for examination
NT **Mental Health and Related Services Act 2000**	Involuntary admission on grounds of mental illness (s14)/mental disturbance (s15); Mental illness (s6) Mentally disturbed (s4)	Request for assessment may be made by a MP or anyone with a genuine interest or concern
TAS **Mental Health Act 1996**	Criteria for detention as involuntary patient (s24) Mental illness (s4)	Involuntary admission via an initial order for up to 72 hours for assessment, a continuing care order or an authorisation for temporary admission
ACT **Mental Health (Treatment and Care) Act 1994**	Powers in relation to detention, restraint etc (s35) Mental illness (s3) Mental dysfunction (undefined)	If a MP believes that a person is mentally ill or is suffering from a mental dysfunction, the person is taken to Canberra Hospital psychiatric unit
VIC **Mental Health Act 1986**	Criteria for involuntary treatment (s8(1)) Mental illness (s8(1A)) Mental disorder (s3)	Anyone in the community over the age of 18 can request that someone be assessed for involuntary treatment, with the recommendation of a MP
NZ **Mental Health (Compulsory Assessment and Treatment) Act 1992**	Compulsory assessment and treatment (ss8–10) Mental disorder (s2(1))	Anyone (including a MP) who believes that a person may be suffering from a mental disorder may apply for an assessment

Psychiatry at a Glance, Sixth Edition. Cornelius Katona, Claudia Cooper, Mary Robertson. © 2016 John Wiley & Sons, Ltd. Published 2016 by John Wiley & Sons, Ltd.
Companion website: www.ataglanceseries.com/psychiatry

Western Australia (WA): A psychiatrist may make a CTO. A CTO is valid for up to three months if within 72 hours it is confirmed by another psychiatrist or authorised MP. The supervising psychiatrist can revoke a CTO.

Northern Territories (NT): A community management plan authorises the involuntary treatment or care of a person in the community. An authorised psychiatric practitioner may make an interim community management order (valid up to 14 days). The MHRT must review the interim order within 14 days. An authorised psychiatric practitioner may suspend a community management order.

Tasmania (TAS): A CTO may be made by two approved MPs who have each separately and within the previous seven days examined the patient. A CTO is valid for up to one year. The MHRT must review a CTO within 28 days.

Australian Capital Territory (ACT): Community care orders are made by the ACT Civil and Administrative Tribunal. A community care order is a form of mental health order and valid for up to six months; it is not age limited.

Victoria (VIC): An authorised psychiatrist may make a CTO. A CTO is valid for up to one year. The authorised psychiatrist may revoke a CTO.

New Zealand (NZ): Wherever possible a CTO is heard and determined by a Family Court judge after examination by a number of MPs who formed the opinion that the person met the criteria set out in the MHA for compulsory treatment. The patient is required to attend and 'accept' treatment in the first month of the CTO and thereafter if a psychiatrist appointed by the MHRT considers that the treatment is in their best interests. The CTO must be reviewed at least every six months.

Forensic sections

NSW: A magistrate, if of the view that a defendant is (or was at the time of the alleged offence) 'developmentally disabled' (not defined) or is suffering from a 'mental illness' (see MHA) or a 'mental condition' (not defined) for which treatment is available in a mental health facility, but is not a 'mentally ill person' within the MHA, can make various procedural or final orders. A final order means that the charge is dismissed and the defendant discharged unconditionally or on condition for assessment and/or treatment.

QLD: A 'forensic order' made by a judge of the Mental Health Court in respect of a forensic patient remains in force until revoked by the MHRT. The MHRT must not revoke a forensic order unless satisfied that the patient does not represent an unacceptable risk to self or others.

SA: 'Supervision orders' include a 'limiting term' cap and can be revoked by the Supreme Court, whereupon the person can be released after taking into account, among other matters, the nature of the person's mental impairment, whether the person is, or would if released be, likely to endanger others, and whether there are adequate resources available for their care in the community.

WA: The Governor may order the release of a person from custody if the Minister, based on a recommendation by the Mental Health Review Board, advises the Governor to do so. However, if a trial judge determines that an accused is unfit and

will not become fit within six months, the judge may quash the indictment (or dismiss the case if there is no indictment) without deciding the guilt or otherwise of the accused and may either release the accused or make a 'custody order' in respect of the accused.

NT: A 'supervision order' (potentially for an indefinite term) must be reviewed every year by the Supreme Court which *must* vary it to a non-custodial supervision order unless satisfied that this would put the safety of the supervised person or the public seriously at risk. The court must consider an appropriate medical report and treatment plan.

TAS: If a person is found unfit for trial and not likely to become fit in 12 months, the court must hold a special hearing. If the person is not found not guilty, or is found not guilty on the grounds of insanity, then the court may make a custodial 'restriction order', a continuing care order or a community treatment order, or the court may release the person conditionally or unconditionally. The patient must be reviewed every 12 months by the Forensic Tribunal, and if determined that the order is no longer necessary, the Supreme Court may discharge or revoke the order.

ACT: The tribunal reviewing an 'order for detention' must take into account: dangerousness/public safety, the nature and extent of the person's mental dysfunction and its likely effect on their future behavior, and the likely sentence of imprisonment had the person been found guilty.

VIC: A 'custodial supervision order' is reviewed by the court and must ordinarily be confirmed or varied to a 'non-custodial supervision order' (which is for an indefinite period). The court must take into account similar matters to those that must be considered in SA.

NZ: The Family Court has principal jurisdiction in mental health matters and oversees offenders who have entered the system of 'compulsory care' but has no jurisdiction in criminal matters affecting patients.

Guardianship (see also Chapter 40 regarding Mental Capacity)

Where a person has a disability that affects their capacity to make informed decisions (e.g. intellectual impairment, mental disorder, brain injury, physical disability or dementia) all jurisdictions allow a legal guardian to be appointed (by a court, board or tribunal). Relevant legislation is:

NSW: Guardianship Act 1987; QLD: Guardianship and Administration Act 2000; SA: Guardianship and Administration Act 1993; WA: Guardianship and Administration Act 1990; NT: Adult Guardianship Act 1988; TAS: Guardianship and Administration Act 1995; ACT: Guardianship and Management of Property Act 1991; VIC: Guardianship and Administration Board Act 1986; NZ: Protection of Personal and Property Rights Act 1988.

Mental Health Review Tribunals

MHRTs conduct mental health inquiries, make and review orders including CTOs, hear appeals and make other decisions about the treatment and care of people with mental illness. They are usually composed of three members: a lawyer (chair), a psychiatrist and another suitably qualified member.

Preparing for Clinical Examinations in Psychiatry

45

Introduction

Objective structured clinical examinations (OSCEs) are now used in most UK medical schools to assess clinical specialities, including psychiatry. An OSCE examination consists of several (usually 16–20) stations with a standard and relatively short time (5–15 minutes) spent on each.

• Sticking to task and time is therefore vital.

• Remember that the marking system is standardised and that stations are distributed across the main topic areas that you should cover.

• A good revision technique is to write some OSCE stations yourselves, preferably in a revision group, and devise your own marking sheet (see our examples in the self-assessment section of this book).

• It is good to practise OSCE scenarios in groups of three, so that one can be the patient, one the candidate and one can assess and give feedback as the examiner.

In this chapter we outline different types of OSCE station and give some practice tips.

Before you start

Read the question carefully, and reread it, taking 10–15 seconds at the beginning (longer than it sounds!) to make sure you are clear what the task is and to think about how to begin. Take note of your role (GP, psychiatrist), and introduce yourself as this.

You could say, '*Hello, Mr John Smith, my name is Dr Jones, a GP at this practice.*' This ensures you are talking to the right patient. Asking the patient to confirm their name, date of birth, occupation etc. at the beginning does nothing to build rapport, so avoid it unless you are specifically asked to do this.

Ask the patient what he or she wants to be called.

Take note of what the patient or relative is expecting. For example, if you have been asked to assess alcohol use or memory in someone who has come about a different matter, saying, '*I understand you're here about your alcohol/memory problem*' could get you off to a bad start!

Start out with a brief, open question: '*How can I help?*'

During the OSCE

• Start with open questions (to which a longer descriptive answer is expected) and move towards closed questions (yes/no answers) as the consultation progresses.

• Don't waste time discussing things that are not relevant to the task. If the question says 'Assess this man's current risk of suicide', you will get marks for asking about his current thoughts, plans and intentions, so refocus and signpost the conversation if it drifts away from the task: '*That sounds like something we certainly need to discuss, but I really want to understand how you feel about x before we move on.*'

• Listen to the patient and ask follow-up questions to clarify any points that are not clear. For example, if they mention that things have been difficult at work or home recently, perhaps the disorder has had an important impact on their work or relationship. If you say, '*I'm sorry to hear that. How have things been difficult?*' you will find out.

• Use language that is understandable to people without a medical degree.

• Acknowledge any distress a patient shows (e.g. '*I'm sorry this is upsetting*').

• Always leave time to summarise back to the patient what has been said. This allows for clarification and a chance for the patient to mention anything important they may have forgotten. Here are some typical tasks requested in OSCE stations and tips on how to address them.

Interview stations

Giving information to a patient or relative, about a diagnosis, treatment or prognosis

• You will not be expected to take a history unless the question specifically tells you so to do.

• Practise succinctly explaining the main psychiatric diagnoses (e.g. schizophrenia, bipolar affective disorder, depression, dementia); try to avoid technical language, or explain any terms you use (e.g. 'tests of kidney function', not 'U&Es').

• Ensure that you first check what the patient/carer knows and a little bit about their particular condition. They want to know about their own illness, not about the condition generally. But don't delay answering their question. So, if they ask, '*What is dementia?*' you can give a general answer and then say that it varies a lot between people, and ask if that sound like the types of difficulty their mother has been having?

• Ask if there are things they particularly want to know, ensure all information is given in small chunks and, after giving each explanation, check if that answers their questions.

• Ensure the actor has a chance to speak; it is not a mini-lecture and people can only take a few pieces of information on board at a time.

• At the end, explain how they can get in touch with someone (care coordinator, GP etc.) in the future and offer to send them leaflets or refer them to appropriate Internet sites (e.g. MIND, Alzheimer's Society) to show you know that they will not remember everything.

Assessing suicide risk

• This is a very common station, so well worth practising.

• If you are asked to assess someone's level of suicide risk after a recent attempt, make sure you elicit:

• the key details of the attempt (Were they alone? Was it planned? How were they discovered? Perceived lethality etc.);

• how they feel about it now (thoughts, plans, intent, mood).

• If asked to assess suicide risk, the number of past attempts and family history are relevant, but don't get bogged down in the past history at the expense of current mental state and the recent attempt.

Psychiatry at a Glance, Sixth Edition. Cornelius Katona, Claudia Cooper, Mary Robertson. © 2016 John Wiley & Sons, Ltd. Published 2016 by John Wiley & Sons, Ltd.
Companion website: www.ataglanceseries.com/psychiatry

• Assess the risk factors for suicide, such as sex, age, depression, alcohol/drug abuse, social support, employment and chronic illness.

Eliciting an aspect of the psychiatric history

• This will be in a very focused area, such as taking an alcohol or illicit substance use history.

Depression

• This will be a station focused on taking a depression history. You will need to cover all the core, cognitive and biological symptoms as well as suicidal intention and a brief past psychiatric history.

• The examiner will be looking for you to exclude differential diagnoses such as bipolar disorder and psychosis.

Eliciting an aspect of the mental state

• Again this will be in a focused area.

• Make sure you do not drift into taking a history. For example, if asked to elicit symptoms of depression, ask about current mood, ability to enjoy life, energy levels, negative cognitions (guilt, hopelessness), biological symptoms etc. Don't ask when they first became depressed.

Video stations

• You may be asked to assess a mental state from a video.

• A good way to practise this is to try to write a mental state for a patient you have seen in a ward round and ask for feedback.

• Make sure you write something for every section, even if there is no abnormality you can see – for example, 'cognition grossly normal' or 'no perceptual abnormality detected'.

• Watch for physical signs (e.g. tremor or other extrapyramidal signs, tics, exophthalmos, evidence of liver disease, tattoos, scars, needle marks, obviously over-/underweight, clothes too big) and abnormal or indicative behaviours, such as crying or poor eye contact.

Pencil and paper stations

• You may be asked to discuss a drug chart or section paper (so make sure you have seen and discussed some during your clinical attachment).

Self-assessment

Objective Structured Clinical Examinations (OSCEs)

Section 1: Assessment and Management

(for answers see p. 116)

Candidate instructions: You are a junior psychiatrist working in A&E. You are asked to assess a 28-year-old woman who took an overdose last night and is now medically fit for discharge. Assess her level of risk.

Instructions for person taking role of patient: You are a 28-year-old woman who has been depressed since the end of your relationship last month. You saw your GP because you felt low all the time, with poor sleep and appetite. He referred you to a psychologist (first appointment next week) and started you on mirtazapine, which you have been taking for a few weeks; it seems to be helping. You have no other past psychiatric history and have never self-harmed before.

You took an overdose of 16 paracetamol tablets last night after an argument with your partner. You still share a house and he brought his new partner back to the house. You took the tablets, which you keep for headaches, while he was upstairs. You wanted to die at the time but afterwards got scared and asked your ex-partner for a lift to the hospital. You had drunk about half a bottle of wine before the argument.

You do not currently have suicidal thoughts. You were angry last night but now feel your partner isn't worth throwing your life away for. Also, your friend Karen has told you to ring her anytime if you feel bad again and you would do this, and you feel better because of this support. You live alone but have a number of friends locally whom you see daily. You have no close family. You currently live with your ex-partner, but he will be moving out soon and you are relieved about this. You work as a receptionist, but have been on sick leave recently.

Instructions for person taking role of examiner: Look at the mark sheet and tick off the points as the candidate covers them.

Section 2: Mental Disorders

(for answers see p. 116)

Candidate instructions: You are a junior doctor working in a psychiatric outpatient clinic. This woman's son has recently been diagnosed by your team with schizophrenia. She would like to discuss this with you.

Instructions for person taking role of patient: Your 23-year-old son has recently been diagnosed with paranoid schizophrenia. Ask the doctor the following questions.

1   What does paranoid schizophrenia mean?
2   He is well now; how likely is he to stay well and what can he and the family do to prevent him having a relapse?
3   He wants to go back to college where he was studying English. Would that be OK?

Instructions for person taking role of examiner: Remain silent for the interview, but at the end of the OSCE ask the candidate to summarise the main risks they have identified.

Section 3: Substance and Alcohol Misuse

(for answers see p. 116)

Candidate instructions: You are an Foundation Year 2 (FY2) working in A&E. A 23-year-old lady who is 24 weeks' pregnant presented with decreased fetal movements but has been discharged by the obstetrician after a normal ultrasound scan. She tells you she doesn't want to leave and feels suicidal. You notice injection marks on her left arm; she also has a black eye. Assess her level of risk if discharged from A&E.

At the end of the OSCE, the examiner will ask you to summarise the main risks you have identified.

Instructions for person taking role of patient: You are 24 weeks' pregnant. You are in a violent relationship with your partner, the father of your unborn child with whom you live. He hit you recently and you have a black eye. You inject street heroin about twice a day and use crack cocaine about once every couple of weeks. You drink about two cans of strong lager a day. You don't know what to do to escape your situation so you go to A&E saying you are worried about your unborn baby, but you've just had a scan saying all is well. You often feel that you don't want to live anymore. You have taken three overdoses in the past. You have thought about taking paracetamol that you have at home but you don't want to hurt your unborn baby so don't think you would do this.

Instructions for person taking role of examiner: Remain silent for the interview, but at the end of the OSCE ask the candidate to summarise the main risks they have identified.

Section 4: Psychiatry of Demographic Groups

(for answers see p. 117)

Candidate instructions: You are an FY2 working in child psychiatry. The mother of an 8-year-old child who has recently been diagnosed with attention-deficit hyperactivity disorder (ADHD) comes to see you. She has some questions for you.

Instructions for person taking role of patient: You are the mother of an 8-year-old child who has recently been diagnosed with attention-deficit hyperactivity disorder (ADHD), and you have some questions for the doctor. Ask him/her:

1   What is ADHD?
2   What treatment is there?
3   When/if medication is mentioned, ask about possible side effects.

Psychiatry at a Glance, Sixth Edition. Cornelius Katona, Claudia Crooper, Mary Robertson. © 2016 John Wiley & Sons, Ltd. Published 2016 by John Wiley & Sons, Ltd.
Companion website: www.ataglanceseries.com/psychiatry

Section 5: The Interface of Psychiatry and Physical Health

(for answers see p. 117)

Candidate instructions: You are a GP. A 75-year-old man comes to see you because he is worried about his memory. Ask him some questions to help you make a diagnosis. Do not formally test cognition.

Instructions for person taking role of patient: You are a 75-year-old man who is worried about his memory. For around the last year you have been finding it harder to think of the right words – for example, you recently forgot the word for a jug. You have noticed yourself becoming more forgetful in the last six months – you forget where you put things (e.g. your glasses) and you recently missed a GP appointment because you forgot to look at your calendar. You have no problems concentrating but often have to reread chapters of a book because you forget the plot. You think the problems are getting gradually worse. A few weeks ago you left the gas on, lit, and only noticed when you came back from the shops. About a month ago, you forgot you were running a bath and flooded the bathroom. You have never lost your way when out. You don't need any help looking after yourself or the home; you do your own laundry, shopping etc., although without a shopping list you would forget what to buy. You sleep well, have a good appetite and have not lost any weight recently. You were widowed several years ago. Your daughter lives close by. You do not feel particularly depressed or anxious. You are an active member of your local Green Party and have a good social life, mainly centred around your friends from this group and ex-army colleagues. You take simvastatin for high cholesterol but otherwise are in very good health. You worked as an air traffic controller before your retirement aged 60.

Instructions for person taking role of examiner: Look at the mark sheet and tick off the points as the candidate covers them.

Section 6: Psychiatric Management

(for answers see p. 117)

Candidate instructions: You are a GP. A woman who was recently diagnosed with bipolar affective disorder has come to see you and wants to discuss her diagnosis. She has some questions about her disorder and her medication (lithium carbonate).

Please answer her questions. You do not need to take a history.

Instructions for person taking role of patient:

Ask the doctor the following questions:

1 You were given a diagnosis of bipolar affective disorder during your recent admission. Ask the doctor what this means.
2 You have been told you need to have blood tests while you are on lithium. Ask what they are for.
3 Ask how you should go about it if you want to stop your tablets.
4 Say to the GP that you are worried that if you tell him/her you have stopped the tablets you will be sectioned again.
5 Ask what you should do if you want to get pregnant.

Instructions for person taking role of examiner: Look at the mark sheet and tick off the points as the candidate covers them.

Extended Matching Questions (EMQs)

For the questions below, each option may be used once, more than once or not at all.

Chapters 1–5: Assessment and management

1. Mental state

a Derealisation
b Compulsion
c Delusion
d Illusion
e Hallucination
f Obsession
g Overvalued idea
h Pseudohallucination
i Rumination

What psychiatric sign is being described in these examples? Choose one option.

1 A man tries unsuccessfully to keep violent, sexual images from entering his head.
2 A 52-year-old man spends over an hour checking the gas is turned out on the stove before leaving the house.
3 A woman describes hearing a voice that frightens her inside her head.
4 A woman complains that she feels as if the world is lifeless, as if made out of cardboard.
5 A man gazing at the sky starts to see the face of a goblin in the clouds.
6 A man is becoming increasingly worried that his neighbours are monitoring him. He sees them out so often it feels like 'more than just a coincidence'. He acknowledges he might be wrong about this, although thinks it unlikely.
7 An anxious man continually reviews the events leading to him losing his job.

2. Delusions

a Delusional perception
b Thought withdrawal
c Delusion of reference
d Grandiose delusion
e Nihilistic delusion
f Folie à deux
g Persecutory delusion
h Somatic passivity

Which delusion is being described in these examples? Choose one option.

1 A man believes the government removes his thoughts.
2 A woman believes she can feel her blood temperature rising and that it must be being controlled using lasers by an outside force.

3 An 84-year-old lady and her learning disabled son are refusing to pay their rent because they believe the council is winding the meter on remotely to extract more money from them.
4 A 34-year-old lady is detained by police for causing a public nuisance. She believes she has been invested with special healing powers and that God has told her she is the next Messiah.
5 A man with depression erroneously believes he has lost all his possessions and his house has been destroyed.
6 A man fled the country after seeing a red car parked outside his house. He was convinced this was a sign left for him by the FBI that they wanted him dead.

Chapters 6–16: Mental disorders

3. Diagnosis

a 1 week
b 2 weeks
c 3 weeks
d 1 month
e 6 months
f 1 year
g 18 months
h No time duration specified

1 ICD-10 requires that symptoms are present for at least _____ for a diagnosis of schizophrenia.
2 DSM-5-TR requires that symptoms are present for at least _____ for a diagnosis of schizophrenia.
3 ICD-10 requires that symptoms are present for at least _____ for a diagnosis of a depressive episode.
4 ICD-10 requires that symptoms are present for at least _____ for a diagnosis of generalised anxiety disorder.
5 ICD-10 requires three panic attacks in _____ for a diagnosis of panic disorder.
6 ICD-10 requires that symptoms are present for at least _____ for a diagnosis of a specific phobia.

4. Anxiety disorders and stress reactions

a Obsessive–compulsive disorder (OCD)
b Post-traumatic stress disorder (PTSD)
c Panic disorder
d Agoraphobia
e Social phobia
f Complicated grief
g Specific phobia
h Acute stress reaction

1 Avoiding crowded places is a common symptom.
2 The phobic disorder most commonly referred to secondary care.
3 Often associated with depersonalisation or derealisation.

Psychiatry at a Glance, Sixth Edition. Cornelius Katona, Claudia Cooper, Mary Robertson. © 2016 John Wiley & Sons, Ltd. Published 2016 by John Wiley & Sons, Ltd.
Companion website: www.ataglanceseries.com/psychiatry

4 A phobic disorder that is equally common in men and women.

5 Disorder with an increased prevalence among those with Tourette's syndrome.

6 Onset is typically rapid (e.g. within hours).

5. Personality disorders

  a Anankastic
  b Narcissistic
  c Avoidant
  d Dependent
  e Dissocial
  f Borderline
  g Paranoid
  h Schizoid
  i Schizotypal

Which personality disorders are described below? Choose one option.

1 Not included as a diagnosis in ICD-10.

2 A middle-aged man is referred by Social Services because his hoarding of newspapers is a fire hazard. He has kept every newspaper he has bought for the last 30 years. They are piled in the kitchen. He is preoccupied by cleanliness, and the flat smells of bleach. He used to work as a picture editor for a newspaper but lost his job because his work was impractically slow.

3 A 72-year-old lady has been unable to cope with life since the death of her husband 10 years ago. She has always hated being alone. She lived with her parents until she married. Her husband made all the decisions and she never disagreed because she did not like upsetting him. She is fit and well but is asking to move to a nursing home.

4 A 28-year-old man presents to A&E after slashing his wrists. He has self-harmed on over 50 previous occasions. He describes chronic feelings of emptiness and feels he doesn't always know who the real he is.

5 A personality disorder that is more common among those with relatives who have schizophrenia.

6 The personality disorder that is most prevalent among male prisoners.

6. Unusual syndromes

  a Fregoli syndrome
  b Capgras syndrome
  c Ekbom's syndrome
  d Cotard's syndrome
  e Folie à deux
  f Othello's syndrome
  g De Clerambault's syndrome
  h Munchausen's syndrome
  i Couvade's syndrome
  j Ganser's syndrome

Which of these syndromes are described below? Choose one option.

1 Symptoms are consciously produced.
2 Also known as delusional parasitosis.
3 Seen in expectant fathers.
4 Usually seen in psychotic depression.
5 Classified as induced delusional disorder in ICD-10.
6 Can be a side effect of Parkinson's disease treatment.

7 May carry an increased risk of violence to members of general public.

Chapters 17–18: Substance and alcohol misuse

7. Substance misuse

  a Alcohol
  b Amphetamines
  c Benzodiazepines
  d Cannabis
  e Cocaine
  f Ecstasy (MDMA)
  g Heroin
  h Khat
  i LSD
  j Solvents

To which drug do these statements most apply? Choose one option.

1 Paradoxical aggression is a known side effect.
2 Methadone replacement is a common treatment.
3 There is good evidence that adolescents using this drug are more likely to develop schizophrenia in adult life.
4 A red rash around the mouth is a common sign of abuse.
5 Deaths from hyponatraemia caused by drinking too much water after taking this drug have been reported.
6 The substance that most commonly causes mild cognitive impairment.

Chapters 19–26: Psychiatry of demographic groups

8. Diagnoses in childhood and early adulthood

  a Birth
  b 3 months
  c Age 2
  d Age 5
  e Age 8
  f Age 15
  g Age 22
  h Age 26

Which of these ages would be the most typical time for the following disorders to be diagnosed? Choose one option.

1 Encopresis
2 Oppositional defiant disorder
3 Attention-deficit and hyperactivity disorder
4 Emotionally unstable personality disorder
5 Bulimia nervosa
6 Anorexia nervosa
7 Autism

9. Epidemiology of psychiatry of demographic groups

  a 0.1%
  b 1%
  c 6%
  d 10%
  e 25%
  f 30%
  g 50%
  h 60%
  i 80%

Which of these most accurately estimates? Choose one option.

1 The percentage of the prison population who have an IQ of 85 or more.
2 The percentage of rough sleepers who use illicit drugs.
3 The percentage of rough sleepers with mental illness.
4 The percentage of women who experience significant depression or anxiety during pregnancy.
5 The percentage of births that are followed by puerperal psychosis.
6 The percentage risk of cardiac malformations in neonates born to mothers taking lithium.

Chapters 27–32: The interface of psychiatry and physical illness

10. Cognitive impairment
a Alzheimer's disease
b Mild cognitive impairment
c Acute confusional state
d Alcohol withdrawal
e Vascular dementia
f Lewy body dementia
g Normal pressure hydrocephalus
h Frontotemporal dementia
i Parkinson's disease dementia
j Depressive disorder

Which of these would be the most likely diagnosis in the following situations? Choose one option.

1 Three-year gradual onset of memory loss. The patient now forgets to eat without prompting. No abnormal findings on physical examination and dementia blood screen. CT head scan shows mild involutional change but no other findings.
2 A patient's husband describes onset in last six months of poor concentration, forgetfulness, apathy and urinary incontinence. You notice a wide-based gait on examination. MRI head scan shows enlarged ventricular system.
3 The patient presents with concerns about her memory, forgetting where she has put things. The forgetfulness dates from the loss of her husband nine months ago. She reports poor sleep and loss of appetite. She is tearful and low in mood with anxiety about her memory loss. Objective clinical cognitive tests are within the normal range.
4 A patient presents with forgetfulness and disorientation to time and place with associated impairment in activities of daily living. Relatives date the onset to a documented cerebrovascular accident two years ago. CT head scan shows a mature infarct in the caudate nucleus and internal capsule.
5 A patient presents with gradual onset of forgetfulness, with a poor memory for recent events. This has not interfered with his daily life, although he now writes a shopping list rather than relying on his memory. Objective clinical cognitive tests are in the borderline range, below those expected given his high educational attainment.
6 A 56-year-old lady is brought to the GP by her husband, who reports a change in her behaviour over the last year. She has become more extrovert, making inappropriate jokes and on one or two occasions acting aggressively towards him. She has no concerns, although when asked did admit to word-finding difficulties. Clinical cognitive tests demonstrated poor performance on verbal fluency and executive functioning.
7 A patient being treated for a urinary tract infection is noted to have poor concentration. Her speech is confused and rambling and she appears to be visually hallucinating. The nurses report fluctuations in her confusion.

11. Psychiatric disorders and physical symptoms and signs
a Somatisation disorder
b Factitious disorder
c Hypochondriacal disorder
d Munchausen disorder by proxy
e Dissociative disorder
f Dysmorphophobia
g Ganser's syndrome
h Depressive disorder
i Panic disorder

Which of these are best described below? Choose one option.

1 Someone with this disorder may typically reply to the question 'What is 2+2?' with the answer 'Five'.
2 A possible differential in a child repeatedly presenting with haematuria of unknown cause.
3 Might typically involve a presentation to A&E with complete memory loss for personal information including name and identity.
4 A patient is discovered to be consciously feigning a left-sided weakness.
5 Often presents first to plastic surgeons.
6 Ten times more common in people with chronic obstructive airways disease.

Chapters 33–44: Psychiatric management

12. Psychological therapies
a Cognitive behavioural therapy (CBT)
b Interpersonal psychotherapy
c Behavioural activation
d Behavioural management therapy
e Dialectical behaviour therapy
f Eye movement desensitisation and reprocessing
g Psychodynamic psychotherapy
h Therapeutic community
i Cognitive analytic therapy
j Person-centred counselling

Which of these are best described below? Choose one option.

1 A residential therapy.
2 A therapy for which transference and counter-transference are key therapeutic tools.
3 Mostly used to treat PTSD.
4 Designed for treatment of borderline (emotionally unstable) personality disorder.
5 A useful intervention in severe dementia, in which the therapy would primarily be conducted with the carer.
6 Focuses on activity scheduling to encourage patients to approach activities that they are avoiding.

13. Treatment of psychosis and depression
a 2 weeks
b 3 weeks
c 4 weeks
d 3 months
e 6 months
f 2 years
g 10 years

1 Risk of relapse is increased significantly if antipsychotics are not continued for _____after recovery from a psychotic episode.

2 Maintenance antidepressant medication after recovery from depressive episode is typically recommended for _____.

3 Antidepressants usually take _____ to manifest their clinical effectiveness.

4 A typical duration of treatment for psychoanalytic psychotherapy is _____ .

5 A typical duration of CBT treatment is _____ .

6 Depot antipsychotic medication is typically administered with a frequency of between once a week and every _____.

14. Treatment in psychiatry
a Antipsychotic medication
b Benzodiazepine
c CBT alone
d Electroconvulsive therapy (ECT)
e Family therapy
f Mood stabiliser
g Psychodynamic psychotherapy
h Selective serotonin reuptake inhibitor (SSRI) and CBT
i SSRI only
j Cholinesterase inhibitor

Which of these would be the most appropriate treatment for the following situations? Choose one option.

1 An 85-year-old lady diagnosed with mild Alzheimer's disease.

2 A 64-year-old man has been severely depressed for several months, and his condition is deteriorating despite treatment with antidepressants. He is very distressed, suicidal and refusing to eat.

3 A 31-year-old mother of a two-month-old baby asks her GP for help. Her GP diagnoses mild depressive disorder.

4 A 28-year-old man with severe OCD. He is no longer able to go to work because it takes him several hours to get dressed every morning as a result of his compulsive rituals.

5 A 34-year-old lady seeks help from her GP. She is concerned that she has problems in intimate relationships due to sexual abuse that she experienced as a child. She feels this is making her very anxious.

6 An 11-year-old boy is brought to the child psychiatry clinic by his mother. She is concerned that he is very distressed and has started to misbehave at school as a result of family difficulties. His father recently moved back home after a period of marital separation.

15. Psychiatry and the English law
a Mental Capacity Act
b Deprivation of Liberty safeguards
c Mental Health Act (MHA), section 2
d MHA, section 3
e MHA, section 5(2)
f MHA, section 17
g MHA, section 37
h MHA, section 58
i MHA, section 135
j MHA, section 136

Which legal act, or section of legal act, is most appropriate to use in these situations? Choose one option.

1 A man who is actively suicidal asks to self-discharge. The medical team contact you, the psychiatry FY2, to ask advice; they need to do something immediately to prevent him leaving.

2 A woman with a known diagnosis of schizophrenia has been shouting at neighbours that they are trying to poison her. When the mental health team visit, she refuses to open the door. They think she needs a psychiatric assessment.

3 You are called to assess a woman with dementia who is refusing potentially life-saving intravenous antibiotics for treatment of cellulitis. She does not believe she is ill.

4 You assess a man with no previously documented psychiatric history who was brought to A&E by his wife. He has threatened to set fire to next door's house because he believes MI5 are using it as a monitoring station. He wants to go home.

5 A consultant psychiatrist treating a man for a psychotic episode under Section 3 of the MHA wants to send him home on leave for a few hours.

6 A 28-year-old woman was arrested after attacking a passer-by, whom she believed was possessed by a demon that was trying to kill her. The courts find her guilty of grievous bodily harm and accept the recommendation that she should be detained in a psychiatric hospital for treatment of a psychotic disorder.

7 A man with moderately severe learning disabilities who is not allowed to leave his group home alone for his own safety persistently bangs on the front door in the morning saying he wants to go for a walk.

Single Best Answer (SBA) Questions

Chapters 1 and 2 (history and examination)

1 A full assessment of a patient newly admitted to a psychiatric unit can be complete without:
   A A full history and mental state examination
   B A risk assessment
   C A physical examination
   D Psychometric testing

Chapter 3 Diagnosis and Classification

2 According to the diagnostic hierarchy, where patients potentially meet criteria for two disorders, precedence should be given to a diagnosis of:
   A Borderline personality disorder rather than depression
   B Generalised anxiety disorder rather than hyperthyroidism
   C Acute psychotic episode rather than dementia
   D Schizophrenia rather than mood disorder

Chapter 4 Risk Assessment and Management

3. Doctors should always break confidentiality if:
   A A victim of domestic abuse refuses help
   B A victim of elder abuse refuses help
   C A patient threatens to kill his cousin
   D A patient admits to regular shoplifting

Chapter 5 Suicide and Deliberate Self-harm

4. Safe management of a person seen in A&E after an overdose must include:
   A At least a brief period of psychiatric admission for assessment
   B A medical assessment
   C An assessment by the Crisis Resolution Team (CRT)
   D A collateral history

Chapter 6 Schizophrenia – Symptoms and Aetiology

5. The most common subtype of schizophrenia is:
   A Paranoid schizophrenia
   B Hebephrenic schizophrenia
   C Catatonic schizophrenia
   D Simple schizophrenia

6. Psychosis is best described as:
   A An illness characterised by symptoms such as depersonalisation and illusions
   B A mild form of schizophrenia
   C Loss of the ability to distinguish reality from fantasy
   D A split personality

Chapter 7 Schizophrenia: Management and Prognosis

7. When initiating antipsychotics in a patient with a new diagnosis of schizophrenia:
   A Consider clozapine
   B Start with a typical antipsychotic
   C Start at lowest recommended dose for your choice of drug
   D Consider that it is often preferable to use depot medication to prevent relapse once well

Chapter 8 Depression

8. First-line treatments for mild depression do not usually include:
   A Antidepressants
   B Self-help group
   C Computer-aided CBT
   D Advice about decreasing alcohol intake

Chapter 9 Bipolar Affective Disorder

9. Bipolar affective disorder is more common in:
   A Men
   B People from lower socioeconomic groups
   C Pregnant women
   D People with a history of sexual abuse

Chapter 10 Stress Reactions (Including Bereavement)

10. An appropriate initial treatment for post-traumatic stress disorder would be:
   A Debriefing
   B Eye movement desensitisation therapy and reprocessing
   C Quetiapine
   D Lorazepam

11. Symptoms that often occur in recently bereaved people without mental illness include:
   A Hearing the voice of the deceased
   B Suicidal intent
   C Agoraphobia
   D Recurrent panic attacks

Chapter 11 Anxiety Disorders

12. First-line treatments for panic disorder do not usually include:
   A CBT
   B SSRIs
   C Benzodiazepines
   D Self-help materials along CBT principles

Psychiatry at a Glance, Sixth Edition. Cornelius Katona, Claudia Cooper, Mary Robertson. © 2016 John Wiley & Sons, Ltd. Published 2016 by John Wiley & Sons, Ltd.
Companion website: www.ataglanceseries.com/psychiatry

Chapter 12 Obsessions and Compulsions

13. A patient tells you he is concerned he may jump in front of a train. He is terrified of doing so, does not want to die but cannot get the thought out of his head. Is this symptom most likely to be?

- **A** Suicidal ideation
- **B** An obsessional impulse
- **C** Anxious rumination
- **D** A compulsion

Chapter 13 Eating Disorders

14. In the treatment of anorexia nervosa, hospitalisation is almost always indicated if:

- **A** There is an absence of insight
- **B** The patient does not comply with treatment
- **C** The patient has a Body Mass Index of below 13.5
- **D** The patient has suicidal ideation

Chapter 14 Personality Disorders

15. Borderline (emotionally unstable) personality disorder:

- **A** Is the most prevalent personality disorder in the general population
- **B** Is usually a lifelong condition
- **C** Is associated with bulimia nervosa
- **D** Can be expected to worsen with age

Chapter 15 Psychosexual Disorders

16. In the context of sexual identity disorders, which of the following is not true?

- **A** Boys who show gender atypical behaviour usually grow up to be homosexual
- **B** Pre-surgery psychotherapy is associated with a favourable outcome to gender reassignment therapy
- **C** Transsexual people believe their biological sex is inappropriate
- **D** Cross-dressing is not associated with sexual excitement

Chapter 16 Unusual Psychiatric Syndromes

17. Munchausen's syndrome is synonymous with:

- **A** Somatisation disorder
- **B** Dissociative disorder
- **C** Hypochondriacal disorder
- **D** Factitious disorder

Chapter 17 Substance Misuse

18. Drugs often used to treat opiate dependence include:

- **A** Buprenorphine
- **B** Bupropion
- **C** Naloxone
- **D** Morphine

Chapter 18 Alcohol Misuse

19. Which of the following is true?

- **A** Alcohol dependence is no longer more common in men
- **B** A quarter of primary care attendees have an alcohol use problem
- **C** The CAGE questionnaire is a useful means of diagnosing alcohol dependence
- **D** Increasing the cost of alcoholic drinks is an effective means of reducing alcohol dependence in a population

Chapters 19 and 20 Child Psychiatry

20. Before the age of 10, girls and boys are equally likely to suffer from:

- **A** Tourette's syndrome
- **B** Autism
- **C** Enuresis
- **D** Depression

21. With regard to autism:

- **A** Onset is usually before nine months
- **B** Around half of patients have normal intelligence
- **C** It is more common in girls
- **D** It is more common in higher social classes

Chapter 21 The Psychiatry of Adolescence

22. Which of the following is not true of a 15-year-old?

- **A** They may consent to a serious operation if a doctor judges they have capacity to do so
- **B** They may be detained under the Mental Health Act
- **C** They may be given treatment that neither they nor their parent consents to if they are made a ward of court and the court agrees it is in their best interests
- **D** They can be detained under the Mental Capacity Act (in England) so long as Deprivation of Liberty Safeguards procedures are followed

Chapter 22 Learning Disability (Mental Retardation)

23. People with mild learning disability:

- **A** Often have sensory impairments
- **B** Rarely live independently
- **C** Are usually diagnosed by three years of age
- **D** Usually have parents with low IQ

Chapter 23 Cross-cultural Psychiatry

24. The prevalence of schizophrenia is higher in African Caribbean people. Possible reasons do not include:

- **A** Higher rates of socioeconomic disadvantage in African Caribbean people living in the UK
- **B** A genetic predisposition to psychosis in African Caribbean people
- **C** The stress of migration
- **D** The stress of racism

Chapter 24 Psychiatry and Social Exclusion

25. Which is true of prisoners with severe mental illness?

- **A** May require treatment in the prison hospital wing under the Mental Health Act
- **B** Can be transferred to a secure psychiatric unit without the consent of the court for urgent treatment
- **C** Are more likely to have a learning disability than people with severe mental illness in the community
- **D** Are less likely to commit suicide than people with severe mental illness in the community because of high levels of observation

Chapter 25 Psychiatry and Female Reproduction

26. Which of the following is true of prescribing psychotropic medication in pregnancy?

- **A** Sertraline and lithium carry similar risks to the foetus
- **B** Prescribing psychotropic medication in pregnancy should always be avoided

C Benzodiazepines are generally safer than antidepressants

D Sodium valproate and carbemazepine are among the most teratogenic psychotropic drugs

Chapter 26 Functional Psychiatric Disorders in Old Age

27. Compared with depression in younger people, an incident case of depression in a 65-year-old man is:

A More likely to be treated

B More likely to have a strong genetic component

C Less likely to be associated with brain imaging abnormalities

D Likely to have a higher risk of mortality

Chapter 27 Psychiatry and Physical Illness

28. Compared with dissociative disorders, somatisation disorders are:

A Less common

B More likely to present with symptoms than clinical signs

C More likely to have complaints that involve the nervous system

D More likely to have symptoms that are deliberately feigned

Chapters 28–30 Neuropsychiatry

29. A single ischaemic cerebrovascular accident (CVA) is unlikely to cause the onset of:

A Tourette's syndrome

B Vascular dementia

C Delirium

D Depression

30. Which of the following endocrine disorders is more likely to present with episodic anxiety than with depression?

A Phaeochromocytoma

B Hypothyroidism

C Hypopituitarism

D Hypocortisolaemia

Chapter 31 Acute Confusional States

31. Useful preventative strategies to avoid delirium on an acute hospital ward do not include:

A Benzodiazepines for poor sleep

B Family photos and other familiar objects around the bed

C Clear signage

D Regular visits from family and friends

Chapter 32 The Dementias

32. In Alzheimer's disease, a treatment associated with beneficial cognitive effects is:

A Electroconvulsive therapy

B Memantine

C Selective serotonin re-uptake inhibitors

D Antipsychotics

Chapter 33 Psychological Therapies

33. Psychodynamic psychotherapy is usually contraindicated in patients with:

A A history of sexual abuse

B Narcissistic personality disorder

C Alcohol dependence

D Psychopathic personality disorder

Chapter 34 Antipsychotics

34. Antipsychotics:

A Are usually given as depot injections to increase adherence

B Usually take four weeks to demonstrate an effect

C Should be continued for ten years after a severe psychotic episode

D If atypical, are commonly associated with metabolic side effects

Chapter 35 Antidepressants

35. Antidepressants are not usually used to treat:

A Anorexia nervosa

B Psychotic depression

C Obsessive–compulsive disorder

D Bulimia nervosa

Chapter 36 Other Psychotropic Drugs

36. Lithium:

A Has a wide therapeutic window

B Must never be prescribed to pregnant women

C Should not be started without a full assessment including liver function tests

D Reduces the risk of suicide

Chapter 37 Electroconvulsive Therapy and Other Treatments

37. Which of these treatments requires no local or general anaesthetic?

A Eye movement desensitisation and reprocessing therapy

B Electroconvulsive therapy (ECT)

C Deep brain stimulation

D Anterior cingulotomy

Chapter 38 Psychiatry in the Community

38. Around 15% of the general population have at some time experienced:

A Mental illness

B Suicidal ideation

C Psychosis

D Personality disorder

Chapter 39 Forensic Psychiatry

38. Shoplifting is not known to be more common than in the general population among people with:

A Substance misuse

B Learning disability

C Emotionally unstable personality disorder

D Generalised anxiety disorder

Chapter 40 Mental Capacity Act

40. The Mental Capacity Act (England and Wales) does not give the legal authority to give the following treatment to a person without capacity to consent:

A An antidepressant to a person with learning disability in a residential home

B Antibiotics to a psychiatric inpatient detained under the Mental Health Act

C Life-saving treatment to a medical inpatient

D Urgent ECT to a psychiatric inpatient detained under the Mental Health Act

Chapter 41 Mental Health Legislation in England and Wales

41. To be detained under a Community Treatment Order:

    A The patient must be detained under Section 2 or 3

    B The approved mental health professional (AMHP) must agree to it

    C The patient must agree to it

    D The patient must be over the age of 18

Chapter 42 Mental Health Legislation in Scotland

42. A Community Treatment Order may be terminated by:

    A The patient's advocate

    B The Mental Welfare Commission

    C The patient

    D A Member of the Scottish Parliament

Chapter 43 Mental Health Legislation in Northern Ireland

43. Which of the following is true of detention under the act?

    A All detained patients are initially admitted for 14 days

    B An Article 4 application must be supported by two doctors' recommendations

    C The patient must agree to it

    D A Form 10 is signed by a doctor and allows detention for a six-month period

Chapter 44 Mental Health Legislation in Australia and New Zealand Australia

44. Which of the following is not a role of the Mental Health Review Tribunal?

    A Conduct mental health inquiries

    B Make and review Community Treatment Orders (CTOs)

    C Hear appeals, and make decisions about the treatment and care of people with a mental illness

    D Assess and determine whether a person has a mental illness

New Zealand

45. The following is true of Community Treatment Orders (CTOs):

    A They must be reviewed every year

    B The patient must attend and accept treatment in the first month

    C They are usually heard and determined by a Mental Health Review Tribunal

    D Examination by a medical practitioner is not an absolute requirement

OSCE Examiner Mark Sheets

( ) represents one mark

Section 1: Assessment and Management
Examiner's mark sheet
( ) Polite and appropriate introduction
( ) Demonstrates empathy
( ) Appropriate use of silence to give time to talk
( ) Responding to verbal and non-verbal cues
( ) Good balance of open and closed questions

Elicit information about recent suicide attempt
( ) Method (paracetamol)
( ) Number of tablets
( ) To what degree it was premeditated (spontaneous, decision to take overdose arose after argument)
( ) Were steps taken to prevent discovery (no, partner was upstairs)
( ) Alcohol taken prior to attempt
( ) Help seeking – asked for lift to hospital

Current mental state
( ) Current suicidal ideation (no)
( ) Why has this changed (angry last night, support of friend)
( ) Ask whether she would feel able to talk to someone if intent returned

Psychiatric history
( ) No past history of self-harm
( ) Recent diagnosis of depression
( ) Adherent to treatment (antidepressants and planning to attend CBT)
( ) Has partially responded to treatment

Social situation: two of:
( ) ( ) Living with ex-partner but he will move out soon; supported by friends with whom in regular contact; work as receptionist, on sick leave recently

Section 2: Mental Disorders
Examiner's mark sheet
( ) Polite and appropriate introduction
( ) Demonstrates empathy
( ) Avoiding technical language
( ) Responding to verbal and non-verbal cues

Question 1
( ) Explanation of psychosis, for example, "people lose the ability to distinguish imagination or fantasy from reality, for example, fears that someone may break into the house may be common, but people with psychosis might believe that someone has broken into their house when they have not"
( ) if symptoms for a month or more…
( ) and not caused by, for example, a physical illness people are given diagnosis paranoid schizophrenia

Question 2
( ) A fifth of people have no further episodes.
Ways to reduce risk of relapse are
( ) taking medication
( ) for at least 2 years
( ) avoiding drug (especially cannabis) and alcohol use
( ) reducing stress
( ) being aware of early signs of relapse so help can be at early stage

Question 3
Answer should encompass
( ) Importance of getting on with life he wants to lead
( ) Ensuring he has good mental health care while at college – for example, can refer to different Early Intervention Service if different town
( ) Thinking about avoiding factors associated with risk of relapse, for example, high stress and drug use

Section 3: Substance and Alcohol Misuse
Examiner's mark sheet
( ) Polite and appropriate introduction
( ) Demonstrates empathy
( ) Responds to verbal and non-verbal cues
( ) Uses open and closed questions appropriately
( ) Listens and responds appropriately

Assesses suicide risk
( ) Elicit current suicidal thoughts
( ) Elicit recent plan to take paracetamol
( ) Elicit no current suicidal intent
( ) Elicit reason for this is not wanting to hurt unborn child
( ) Ask who (if anyone) she could contact/tell if thoughts returned

Substance misuse
( ) Explore reason for injection marks sensitively
( ) ( ) history of heroin use (two of following: frequency, methods of use (e.g. injecting)), whether sharing needles and if using sterilised needles, injection sites used) e.g. arm, groin)), whether sought or receiving treatment
( ) Cocaine
( ) Cannabis
( ) Alcohol history

Social situation
( ) Elicit reason for black eye (physical abuse from partner)
( ) History of abuse including frequency and…
( ) Severity
( ) Elicit that partner also uses drugs
At the end of the OSCE, the examiner asks you to summarise the main risks:
( ) Suicidal thoughts and recent plan but no current intent
( ) Physical abuse (risk to mother and unborn child)

Psychiatry at a Glance, Sixth Edition. Cornelius Katona, Claudia Cooper, Mary Robertson. © 2016 John Wiley & Sons, Ltd. Published 2016 by John Wiley & Sons, Ltd.
Companion website: www.ataglanceseries.com/psychiatry

( ) Risks from injecting heroin (you might mention (but not needed for mark) hepatitis B and C, HIV, risk of DVT from injecting in groin, especially in pregnancy)

( ) Risks to unborn child from substance use (you might mention (but not needed for mark) risks from impurities in street heroin, of withdrawal syndrome at birth; cocaine is a vasoconstrictor that can affect placenta; from alcohol)

( ) Risks to newborn (you might mention (but not needed for mark) violence in home, drug taking, impact of maternal depression on bonding)

Section 4: Psychiatry of Demographic Groups

Examiner's mark sheet

( ) Polite and appropriate introduction
( ) Demonstrates empathy
( ) Responds to verbal and non-verbal cues
( ) Uses open and closed questions appropriately
( ) Listens and responds appropriately

Question 1

( ) ( ) ( ) ( ) Describes four core symptoms in way understandable to mother: short attention span; easily distracted; overactive; acts impulsively

( ) Symptoms cause difficulties – for example, with school work or in social relationships

( ) Say it happens in more than one place, for example, home and school

Question 2

( ) Methylphenidate

( ) Explain there are also some psychological treatments where a psychologist or other professional talks to parent about helpful ways to manage behaviour

Question 3

( ) Decreased appetite/weight loss
( ) Difficulty sleeping
( ) Feeling agitated or anxious
( ) Explain that side effects would be monitored and reassure that drug would only be used if benefits outweighed difficulties

Section 5: The Interface of Psychiatry and Physical Health

Examiner's mark sheet

( ) Polite and appropriate introduction
( ) Demonstrates empathy
( ) Responds to verbal and non-verbal cues
( ) Uses open and closed questions appropriately
( ) Listens and responds appropriately

Elicits history of memory problems

( ) Forgetfulness for about six months
( ) Word-finding difficulties for a year
( ) Gradual worsening of symptoms

( ) No problems with concentration
( ) ( ) Two of: forgetting appointments, where put things, rereading chapters of book, forgets what to buy without shopping list

Ask about impact on daily life

( ) Leaving the gas on
( ) Flooding the bathroom
( ) No history of getting lost or being disorientated when out
( ) Fully self-caring

Questions to screen for possible causes of memory loss

( ) Elicit whether low in mood
( ) Ask about sleep
( ) Ask about appetite and recent loss of weight
( ) Ask about physical health
( ) Ask about current medication

Section 6: Psychiatric Management

Examiner's mark sheet

( ) Polite and appropriate introduction
( ) Demonstrates empathy
( ) Use of appropriate language (avoiding excessive technical language and explaining terms used)
( ) Ascertained existing level of knowledge
( ) Asks patient for feedback about whether information understandable/answered the question
( ) Responds to verbal and non-verbal cues
( ) Offers leaflets or further source of information

Question 1

( ) Episodic illness, well between episodes
( ) Mood disorder
( ) Depressive episodes
( ) Manic episodes (increased mood, feelings of increased abilities or esteem, decreased sleep, reckless or impulsive behaviour)

Question 2

( ) To ensure safe but adequate levels of lithium
( ) To detect any side effects (renal/thyroid problems) so they can be managed or medication stopped

Questions 3 and 4

( ) Advise to consult GP if concerns about medication
( ) Consider other medication OR reducing gradually
( ) Would not section someone who was well because they had stopped taking medication
( ) More likely to have a further episode if stop medication
( ) If mental health, safety or safety of others serious concern and refusing treatment, would be assessed under Mental Health Act

Question 5

( ) Talk to doctor as early as possible, **before trying to conceive**
( ) Potential risk to unborn child from lithium
( ) Need to balance risks from medication against need to stay well

Answers to EMQs

1 Mental state
1 f (obsessional images)
2 b
3 h
4 a
5 d
6 g
7 i

2 Delusions
1 b
2 h
3 f
4 d
5 e
6 a

3 Diagnosis
1 d
2 e
3 b
4 c
5 c
6 h

4 Anxiety disorders and stress reactions
1 d
2 d
3 c
4 f
5 a
6 h

5 Personality disorders
1 b
2 a
3 d
4 f
5 i
6 e

6 Unusual syndromes
1 h
2 c
3 i
4 d
5 e
6 f
7 a (the patient believes that their persecutors are taking the form of other people so may be aggressive to a member of the public they believe to be their persecutor in disguise)

7 Substance and alcohol misuse
1 c (see Chapter 36)
2 g
3 d
4 j
5 f
6 a

8 Diagnoses in childhood and early adulthood
1 d
2 e
3 e
4 h
5 g
6 f
7 c

9 Epidemiology of psychiatry of demographic groups
1 g
2 g
3 h
4 d
5 a
6 c

10 Cognitive impairment
1 a
2 g
3 j
4 e
5 b
6 h
7 c

11 Psychiatric disorders and physical symptoms and signs
1 1 g
2 d
3 e
4 b
5 f
6 i (see Chapter 11, aetiology section)

12 Psychological therapies
1 h
2 g
3 f
4 e
5 d
6 c

Psychiatry at a Glance, Sixth Edition. Cornelius Katona, Claudia Cooper, Mary Robertson. © 2016 John Wiley & Sons, Ltd. Published 2016 by John Wiley & Sons, Ltd.
Companion website: www.ataglanceseries.com/psychiatry

13 Treatment of psychosis and depression

1 f
2 e
3 c
4 g
5 d
6 c

14 Treatment in psychiatry

1 j
2 d
3 c
4 h
5 g
6 e

15 Psychiatry and the English law

1 e
2 i
3 a
4 c
5 f
6 g
7 b

Answers to Single Best Answer (SBA) Questions

Chapters 1 and 2 (history and examination)

1 D; psychometric testing not administered routinely.

Chapter 3 Diagnosis and Classification

2. D; psychotic disorders take precedence over mood disorders.

Chapter 4 Risk Assessment and Management

3. C; there is always a duty when you are made aware of a specific risk to a named indvidual. For A and B, whether to do so would depend on whether the victim had capacity to make decision to refuse help. For D, there is a duty to disclose information that may help prevent or detect serious crime, but not all crime.

Chapter 5 Suicide and Deliberate Self-harm

4. B; all may be useful, but only B is essential in all cases. Patients may underestimate or not disclose the full extent of their overdose.

Chapter 6 Schizophrenia – Symptoms and Aetiology

5. A.

6. C; note it is hallucinations, not illusions, that are characteristic of psychosis.

Chapter 7 Schizophrenia: Management and Prognosis

7. C; clozapine is only used when two other antipsychotics have failed because of side effects (p. 17); depot is only used where specifically indicated (e.g. because of patient preference or very poor adherence; NICE recommends commencing new patients on an atypical antipsychotic.

Chapter 8 Depression

8. A; antidepressants are generally only recommended for moderate and severe depression.

Chapter 9 Bipolar Affective Disorder

9. D; it is more common in women, with high rates postpartum but not during pregnancy, and in higher socioeconomic groups.

Chapter 10 Stress Reactions (Including Bereavement)

10. B (p. 22).

11. A (p. 22).

Chapter 11 Anxiety Disorders

12. C; benzodiazepines are not recommended.

Chapter 12 Obsessions and Compulsions

13. B; it is egodystonic (the thought is unwelcome and recognised as alien; it is not what he thinks).

Chapter 13 Eating Disorders

14. C.

Chapter 14 Personality Disorders

15. C.

Chapter 15 Psychosexual Disorders

16. A; they usually grow up to be heterosexual.

Chapter 16 Unusual Psychiatric Syndromes

17. D (p. 34).

Chapter 17 Substance Misuse

18. A.

Chapter 18 Alcohol Misuse

19. D; not the CAGE is a useful screening, not diagnostic, test.

Chapters 19 and 20 Child Psychiatry

20. D (see Chapter 19).

21. D (p. 48).

Chapter 21 The Psychiatry of Adolescence

22. D (see Chapter 40; the Mental Capacity Act applies to those aged 18 and over).

Chapter 22 Learning Disability (Mental Retardation)

23. D.

Psychiatry at a Glance, Sixth Edition. Cornelius Katona, Claudia Cooper, Mary Robertson. © 2016 John Wiley & Sons, Ltd. Published 2016 by John Wiley & Sons, Ltd.
Companion website: www.ataglanceseries.com/psychiatry

Chapter 23 Cross-cultural Psychiatry

24. B; *this cannot be true, because rates of schizophrenia in the Caribbean are similar to those in the UK among the indigenous populations.*

Chapter 24 Psychiatry and Social Exclusion

25. C; *treatment under the Mental Health Act may not be given in prison; transfer always requires court approval; prisoners with mental illness are at high risk of suicide.*

Chapter 25 Psychiatry and Female Reproduction

26. D; *the risks of prescribing and not prescribing need to be carefully weighed; lithium is more likely to be teratogenic than sertraline.*

Chapter 26 Functional Psychiatric Disorders in Old Age

27. D; *incident depression in older age is more likely to be associated with brain imaging abnormalities, less likely to be associated with a positive family history, and less likely to be treated compared with depression in a younger person.*

Chapter 27 Psychiatry and Physical Illness

28. B; *They are more common than dissociative disorders; dissociative disorders generally involve the nervous system; in neither disorder are symptoms deliberately feigned; if so, factitious disorder would be the correct diagnosis.*

Chapters 28–30 Neuropsychiatry

29. A; *the others are more common after CVA.*

30. A.

Chapter 31 Acute Confusional States

31. A; *benzodiazepines can contribute to or cause confusion.*

Chapter 32 The Dementias

32. B (pp. 74); *note that antipsychotic use is associated with cognitive decline.*

Chapter 33 Psychological Therapies

33. C; *it is often used as a treatment for the others. It is important that substance misuse problems are under control before initiating psychodynamic psychotherapy because exposing unconscious conflicts can increase stress in the short term and this could lead to increased substance misuse as an unhelpful coping strategy.*

Chapter 34 Antipsychotics

34. D; *most authorities recommend continuing for 2–5 years after a psychotic episode; they generally demonstrate some effect within a week; they are usually taken orally.*

Chapter 35 Antidepressants

35. A.

Chapter 36: Other Psychotropic Drugs

36. D (page 85); *it is teratogenic so female patients should always be advised to consult their doctor if planning a pregnancy because usually they will be changed to safer medication; sometimes patient and doctor decide the risks of stopping (relapse with increased risk of self-harm, accidents and stress) outweigh those of continuing to take it when pregnant.*

Chapter 37: Electroconvulsive Therapy and Other Treatments

37. A (see also Chapter 33).

Chapter 38: Psychiatry in the Community

38. B; *Psychosis (<1%) and personality disorder (5%) are less common; mental illness is more common (25%); see Chapter 38.*

Chapter 39: Forensic Psychiatry

39. D.

Chapter 40: Mental Capacity Act

40. D; *if a patient is detained under the MHA they receive psychiatric treatment under it.*

Chapter 41: Mental Health Act (England and Wales)

41. B.

Chapter 42: Mental Health Legislation in Scotland

42. B.

Chapter 43: Mental Health Legislation in Northern Ireland

43. D.

Chapter 44: Mental Health Legislation in Australia and New Zealand

44. D.

45. B.

Further Reading

Chapters 1–3

American Psychiatric Association (APA) (2013) *Diagnostic and Statistical Manual of Mental Disorder*, 5th edn text revision, APA, Washington, DC.

Kendell, R.E. (2001) The distinction between mental and physical illness. *British Journal of Psychiatry*, 178, 490–493.

Maj, M. (2005) 'Psychiatric comorbidity': an artefact of current diagnostic systems? *British Journal of Psychiatry*, 186, 182–184.

Oyebode F. (2008) *Sims' Symptoms in the Mind: An Introduction to Descriptive Psychopathology*, 4th edn, Saunders Elsevier.

WHO (2002) *The ICD-10 Classification of Mental and Behavioural Disorders*, World Health Organization, Geneva, http//www.who.int/classifications/apps/icd/icd10online (accessed 16 February, 2012).

Chapter 4

Friedman, R.A. (2006) Violence and mental illness – how strong is the link? *New England Journal of Medicine*, 355, 2064–2066.

Royal College of Psychiatrists (2008) Rethinking Risk to Others in Mental Health Services, http://www.rcpsych.ac.uk/files/pdfversion/CR150.pdf (accessed 16 February, 2012).

Chapter 5

Broadhurst, M. and Gill, P. (2007) Repeated self-injury from a liaison psychiatry perspective. *Advances in Psychiatric Treatment*, 13, 228–235.

Department of Health (2011) Consultation on Preventing Suicide in England, http://www.dh.gov.uk/prod_consum_dh/groups/dh_digitalassets/documents/digitalasset/dh_128463.pdf (accessed 16 February, 2012).

Fagin, L. (2006) Repeated self-injury: perspectives from general psychiatry. *Advances in Psychiatric Treatment*, 12, 193–201.

National Confidential Inquiry (NCI) into Suicide and Homicide by People with Mental Illness (2006) Inquiry Reports. NCI: Manchester, http://www.medicine.manchester.ac.uk/ mentalhealth/research/suicide/prevention/nci/inquiry_reports (accessed 16 February, 2012).

National Institute for Clinical Excellence (NICE) (2004) *Self-harm: The Short-term Physical and Psychological Management and Secondary Prevention of Self-harm in Primary and Secondary Care*, NICE, London, http://www. nice.org.uk/CG16 (accessed 16 February 2012).

Chapters 6 and 7

Davies, E.J. (2007) Developmental aspects of schizophrenia and related disorders: possible implications for treatment strategies. *Advances in Psychiatric Treatment*, 13, 384–391.

McGlashan, T.H. (2005) Early detection and intervention in psychosis: an ethical paradigm shift. *British Journal of Psychiatry*, 187, s113–s115.

NICE (2014) *Psychosis and schizophrenia in adults: treatment and management*, NICE, London, https://www.nice.org.uk/guidance/cg178 (accessed 4 March 2015).

Paparelli, A., Di Forti, M., Morrison, P.D. and Murray, R.M. (2011) Drug-induced psychosis: how to avoid star gazing in schizophrenia research by looking at more obvious sources of light. *Frontiers in Behavioural Neuroscience*, 17 January, doi: 10.3389/fnbeh.2011.00001.

Chapter 8

Katona, C., Peveler, R., Dowrick, C. *et al.* (2005) Pain symptoms in depression: definition and clinical significance. *Clinical Medicine*, 5 (4), 390–395.

Langlands, R.L., Jorm, A.F., Kelly, C.M. and Kitchener, B.A. (2008) First aid for depression: a Delphi consensus study with consumers, carers and clinicians. *Journal of Affective Disorders*, 105, 157–165.

NICE (2009) *Depression: The Treatment and Management of Depression in Adults*, NICE, London, http://www.nice.org.uk/CG90 (accessed 16 February, 2012).

Wolpert, L. (1998) *Malignant Sadness*, Faber, London.

Chapter 9

Angst, J. (2007) The bipolar spectrum. *British Journal of Psychiatry*, 190, 189–191.

Benazzi, F. (2007) Bipolar II disorder: epidemiology, diagnosis and management. *CNS Drugs*, 21(9), 727–740.

Spanemberg, L., Massuda, R., Lovato, L. *et al.* (2011) Pharmacological treatment of bipolar depression: qualitative systematic review of double-blind randomized clinical trials, *Psychiatric Quarterly*, 17 83 (2), 161–175.

Chapter 10

Adshead, G. and Ferris, S. (2007) Treatment of victims of trauma. *Advances in Psychiatric Treatment*, 13, 358–368.

Bisson, J.I. (2007) Post-traumatic stress disorder. *British Medical Journal*, 334, 789–793.

Frueh, B.C., Buckley, T.C., Cusack, K.J. *et al.* (2004) Cognitive–behavioral treatment for PTSD among people with severe mental illness: a proposed treatment model. *Journal of Psychiatric Practice*, 10 (1), 26–38.

NICE (2006) *Post-traumatic Stress Disorder (PTSD): The Management of PTSD in Adults and Children in Primary and Secondary Care*, NICE, London, http://www.nice.org.uk/ CG26 (accessed 16 February, 2012)

Vanderwerker, L.C., Jacobs, S.C., Parkes, C.M. and Prigerson, H.G. (2006) An exploration of associations between separation anxiety in childhood and complicated grief in later life. *Journal of Nervous and Mental Disease*, 194 (2), 121–123.

Psychiatry at a Glance, Sixth Edition. Cornelius Katona, Claudia Cooper, Mary Robertson. © 2016 John Wiley & Sons, Ltd. Published 2016 by John Wiley & Sons, Ltd.
Companion website: www.ataglanceseries.com/psychiatry

Chapter 11

Fricchione, G. (2004) Generalised anxiety disorder. *New England Journal of Medicine*, 351, 675–682.

Katon, W.J. (2006) Panic disorder. *New England Journal of Medicine*, 354, 2360–2367.

NICE (2011) *Generalised Anxiety Disorder and Panic Disorder (With or Without Agoraphobia) in Adults*, NICE, London, http://www.nice.org.uk/CG113 (accessed 16 February, 2012).

Schneier, F.R. (2006) Social anxiety disorder. *New England Journal of Medicine*, 355, 1029–1036.

Chapter 12

Bloch M.H. *et al.* (2013) Long-term outcome in adults with Obsessive-Compulsive Disorder. *Depress Anxiety* 30 (8), 716–722.

Chang K. *et al.* (2015) Clinical evaluation of youth with Paediatric Acute -onset Neuropsychiatric Syndrome (PANS): Recommendations from the 2013 PANS Consensus Conference. *J Child Adolesc Psychopharmacology* February 25 (1) 3–13.

Goodman W.K. *et al.* (2014) Obsessive-Compulsive Disorder. *Psych Clin North Am* 37 (3), 257–267.

Leckman, J.F., Rauch, S.L. and Mataix-Cols, D. (2007) Symptom dimensions in obsessive-compulsive disorder: implications for the DSM-V. *CNS Spectrums*, 12(5), 376–387, 400.

Macerello A., Martino D. (2013) Paediatric Autoimmune Neuropsyciatric Disorders Associated with Streptococcus (PANDAS): an evolving concept. *Tremor Other Hyperkinetic Mov* (NY) September 25 (3) pll:tre 03: 167-4158-7.

Murphy T.K. *et al.* (2015) Pediatric Acute-onset Neuropsychiatric Syndrome. *Psychiatric Clin North Am* 37 (3), 353–374.

NICE (2006) *Obsessive-Compulsive Disorder: Core Interventions in the Treatment of Obsessive-Compulsive Disorder and Body Dysmorphic Disorder*, NICE, London, http://nice.org.uk/ CG31 (accessed 4 March 2015).

Pauls D.L. *et al.* (2014) Obsessive - Compulsive Disorder: an integration of genetic and neurobiological perspectives. *Nat Rev Neurosci* 15 (6), 410–424.

Simpson, H.B. (2010) Pharmacological treatment of obsessive-compulsive disorder. *Current Topics in Behavioral Neurosciences*, 2, 527–543.

Chapter 13

Fitzpatrick, K.K. and Lock, J. (2011) Anorexia Nervosa. *Clinical Evidence* (online), April 11, pii: 1011.

Hudson, J.I., Hiripi, E., Pope, H.G. and Kessler, R. C. (2007) The prevalence and correlates of eating disorders in the National Comorbidity Survey replication. *Biological Psychiatry*, 1, 61 (3), 348–358.

NICE (2004) *Eating Disorders: Core Interventions in the Treatment and Management of Anorexia Nervosa, Bulimia Nervosa and Related Eating Disorders*, NICE, London, http://www.nice.org.uk/CG9.

Treasure, J. and Schmidt, U. (2005) Anorexia nervosa. *Clinical Evidence*. December (14), 1140–1148.

Chapter 14

Dixon-Gordon, K.L., Turner, B.J. and Chapman, A.L. (2011) Psychotherapy for personality disorders. *International Review of Psychiatry*, 23 (3), 282–302.

Howells, K., Krishnan, G. and Daffern, M. (2007) Challenges in the treatment of dangerous and severe personality disorder. *Advances in Psychiatric Treatment*, 13, 325–332.

Paris, J. (2011) Pharmacological treatments for personality disorders. *International Review of Psychiatry*, 23 (3), 303–309.

Tyrer, P., Coombs, N., Ibrahimi, F. *et al.* (2007) Critical developments in the assessment of personality disorder. *British Journal of Psychiatry*, May, 49 (Suppl.), s51–s59.

Chapter 15

Lindau, S.T., Schumm, L.P., Laumann, E.O. *et al.* (2007) A study of sexuality and health among older adults in the United States. *New England Journal of Medicine*, 357, 762–774.

Meston, C.M. and Bradford, A. (2007) Sexual dysfunctions in women. *Annual Review of Clinical Psychology*, 3, 233– 256.

Wylie, K. (2008) Erectile dysfunction. *Advances in Psychosomatic Medicine*, 29, 33–49.

Chapter 16

Asher, R. (1951) Munchausen's syndrome. *Lancet*, i, 339–341.

Enoch, M.D. and Trethowan, W. (1991) *Uncommon Psychiatric Syndromes*, Butterworth Heinemann, Oxford.

Lepping, P., Russell, P. and Freudenmann, R.W. (2007) Antipsychotic treatment of primary delusional parasitosis: systematic review. *British Journal of Psychiatry*, 191, 198–205.

Chapters 17 and 18

Ball, D. (2004) Genetic approaches to alcohol dependence. *British Journal of Psychiatry*, 185, 449–451.

Department of Health (England) and the devolved administrations (2007) *Drug Misuse and Dependence: UK Guidelines on Clinical Management*, Department of Health (England), the Scottish Government, Welsh Assembly Government and Northern Ireland Executive, London.

Luty, J. (2006) What works in alcohol use disorders? *Advances in Psychiatric Treatment*, 12, 13–22.

NICE (2010) *Alcohol-Use Disorders: Preventing Harmful Drinking*, NICE, London, http://www.nice.org.uk/PH24, (accessed 16 February, 2012).

Seivewright, N., McMahon, C. and Egleston, P. (2005) Stimulant use still going strong: revisited … misuse of amphetamines and related drugs. *Advances in Psychiatric Treatment*, 11 (4), 262–269.

Chapters 19–21

Arnold L.E. *et al.* (2015) Effect of treatment modality on long-term outcomes in ADHD: a systematic review. *PLoS One* 25 (2): February 25 (epub ahead of print).

Bushra, H. (2007) Anti-social adolescents conduct disorder: a review. *Journal of Community Practice*, 80 (7), 38–40.

Doyle-Thomas K.A. *et al.* (2015) Atypical brain connectivity during rest in ASD. *Annals Neurol* February 23 (epub ahead of print).

Eapen, V. (2011) Genetic basis of autism: is there a way forward? *Current Opinion in Psychiatry*, 24, 226–236.

Eapen V. and Crnec R. (2014) DSM 5 and child psychiatric disorders: What has changed? What is new? *Asian J Psychiatry*, 11, 114–118.

Fabiano G.A. *et al.* (2015) A systematic review of meta-analyses of psychosocial treatment for AttentionDeficit/Hyperactivity Disorder. 18 (1), 77–97.

Friedman, R.A. (2006) Uncovering an epidemic – screening for mental illness in teens. *New England Journal of Medicine*, 355, 2717–2719.

Gawrilow C. *et al.* (2014) Hypereactivity and Motoric Activity in ADHD: characterization, Assesment, and Intervention. *Front Psychiatry* November 28, 5: 171 doi:10.3389/fpsyt.2014.00171.eC.

Gentile, S. (2011) Clinical usefulness of second-generation antipsychotics in treating children and adolescents diagnosed with bipolar or schizophrenic disorders. *Pediatric Drugs*, 13 (5), 291–302.

Jeste S.S. *et al.* (2015) Electroencephalogical biomarkers of diagnosis and outcome in Neurodevelopmental Dsorders. *Curr Opin Neurology* February 23, (epub ahead of print).

Jo H. *et al.* (2015) Age at onset of Autistic Spectrum Disorder (ASD), Diagnosis by Race, Ethnicity and primary household language among children with special health care needs. US 2009–2010. *Maternal Child Health J.* February 21 (epub ahead of print).

NICE (2013) *Depression in Children and Young People: Identification and Management in Primary, Community and Secondary Care*, http://www.nice.org.uk/CG28 (accessed 4 March 2015).

NICE (2008) *Attention Deficit Hyperactivity Disorder: Diagnosis and Management of ADHD in Children, Young People and Adults*, NICE, London, http://www.nice.org.uk/CG72 (accessed 4 March 2015).

Ramdvedt B.E. *et al.* (2013) Clinical gains from including both dextroamphetamine and methylphenidate in stimulant trials. *J Child Adolesc Psychopharmacol* 23 (9), 597–604.

Thapar, A., Langley, K., Asherson, P. and Gill, M. (2007) Gene-environment interplay in attention-deficit hyperactivity disorder and the importance of a developmental perspective. *British Journal of Psychiatry*, 190, 1–3.

Chapter 22

Gallagher, A. and Hallahan, B. (2011) Fragile X-associated disorders: a clinical overview. *Journal of Neurology*. 2012(259), 401–413.

Hassiotis, A. and Hall, I. (2004) Behavioural and cognitive-behavioural interventions for outwardly-directed aggressive behaviour in people with learning disabilities. *Cochrane Database of Systematic Reviews (Online)*, 18 (4), CD003406.

Kwok, H. and Cheung, P.W. (2007) Co-morbidity of psychiatric disorder and medical illness in people with intellectual disabilities. *Current Opinion in Psychiatry*, 20, 443–449.

Chapter 23

Bhugra, D. and Mastrogianni, A. (2004) Globalisation and mental disorders: overview with relation to depression. *British Journal of Psychiatry*, 184, 10–20.

Morgan, C. and Fearon, P. (2007) Social experience and psychosis insights from studies of migrant and ethnic minority groups. *Epidemiologia e Psichiatria Sociale*, 16 (2), 118–123.

Vikash, R., Chaudhury, S., Sukumaran, S. *et al.* (2008) Transcultural psychiatry. *Industrial Psychiatry Journal*, 17, 4–20.

Chapter 24

Fazel, M., Wheeler, J. and Danesh, J. (2005) Prevalence of serious mental disorder in 7000 refugees resettled in western countries: a systematic review. *Lancet*, 365 (9467), 1309–1314.

Grenier, P. (1996) *Still Dying for a Home*, Crisis, London.

Killaspy, H., Ritchie, C., Greer, E. and Robertson, M. (2004) Treating the homeless mentally ill: does a designated inpatient facility improve outcome? *Journal of Mental Health*, 13, 593–599.

Robjant, K., Hassan, R. and Katona, C. (2009) Mental health implications of detaining asylum seekers: a systematic review. *British Journal of Psychiatry* 194, 306–312.

Royal College of Psychiatrists (2006) Improving Services for Refugees and Asylum Seekers: Position Statement. http://www.rcpsych.ac.uk/docs/Refugee%20asylum%20seeker%20consensus%20final.doc (accessed 16 February, 2012).

Chapter 25

Boath, E., Bradley, E. and Henshaw, C. (2005) The prevention of postnatal depression: a narrative systematic review. *Journal of Psychosomatic Obstetrics Gynaecology*, 26 (3), 185–192.

Day, E. and George, S. (2005) Management of drug misuse in pregnancy. *Advances in Psychiatric Treatment*, 11, 253–261.

Doucet, S., Jones, I., Letourneau, N. *et al.* (2011) Interventions for the prevention and treatment of postpartum psychosis: a systematic review. *Archives of Women's Mental Health*, 14 (2), 89–98.

Kohen, D. (2004) Psychotropic medication in pregnancy. *Advances in Psychiatric Treatment*, 10, 59–66.

Chapter 26

Alexopoulos, G.S. (2006) The vascular depression hypothesis: 10 years later. *Biological Psychiatry*, 60 (12), 1304–1305.

Iglewicz, A., Meeks, T.W., Jeste, D.V. (2011) New wine in old bottle: late-life psychosis. *Psychiatric Clinics of North America*, 34 (2), 295–318.

Karim, S. and Byrne, E.J. (2005) Treatment of psychosis in elderly people. *Advances in Psychiatric Treatment*, 11, 286–296.

Katona, C. and Katona, C. (2010) Current challenges faced by clinicians in managing late-life depression: what can be learnt from the recent evidence base? *Mind and Brain, the Journal of Psychiatry* 1, 35–41.

Nelson, J.C., Delucchi, K. and Schneider, L.S. (2008) Anxiety does not predict response to antidepressant treatment in late life depression: results of a meta-analysis. *International Journal of Geriatric Psychiatry*, 24, 539–544.

Chapter 27

Guthrie, E. (2006) Psychological treatments in liaison psychiatry: the evidence base. *Clinical Medicine*, 6, 544–547.

Leentjens, A.F., Rundell, J.R., Diefenbacher, A. *et al.* (2011) Psychosomatic medicine and consultation-liaison psychiatry: scope of practice, processes, and competencies for psychiatrists or psychosomatic medicine specialists. A consensus statement of the European Association of Consultation-Liaison Psychiatry and the Academy of Psychosomatic Medicine. *Psychosomatics*, 52 (1), 19–25.

Owens, C. and Dein, S. (2006) Conversion disorder: the modern hysteria. *Advances in Psychiatric Treatment*, 12, 152–157.

Spence, S.A. (2006) All in the mind? The neural correlates of unexplained physical symptoms. *Advances in Psychiatric Treatment*, 12, 349–358.

Chapters 28–30

Butler, R. (2006) Prion diseases in humans: an update. *British Journal of Psychiatry*, 189, 295–296.

Dilley, M. and Fleminger, S. (2006) Advances in neuropsychiatry: clinical implications. *Advances in Psychiatric Treatment*, 12, 23–34.

Freeman, M., Patel, V., Collins, P.Y. and Bertolote, J. (2005) Integrating mental health in global initiatives for HIV/AIDS. *British Journal of Psychiatry*, 187, 1–3.

Pauls D.L. *et al.* (2014) The inheritance of Tourette Syndrome: a review. *J Obs Comp Related Disord*, 3 (4), 380–385.

Robertson M.M. (2014a) Movement Disorders: Tourette Syndrome – beyond swearing and sex? *Nature Reviews Neurology*, January 10 (1) 6–8.

Robertson M.M. (2014b) A personal 35 year perspective on Gilles de la Tourette Syndrome: prevalence, phenomenology, comorbidities and coexistent psychopathologies. *Lancet Psychiatry*, 2 (1), 68–87.

Robertson M.M. (2014c) A personal 35 year perspective on Gilles de la Tourette Syndrome: assessment, investigations and management. *Lancet Psychiatry*, 2 (1), 88–104.

Robertson M.M., Cavanna A.E. and Eapen V. (2014) Gilles de la Tourette syndrome and disruptive behavior disorders: prevalence, associations and explanation of the relationships. *The Journal of Neuropsychiatry and Clinical Neurosciences*, 2014. August27. doi. 10.1176/appi.neuropsych.13050112 (epub).

Robertson M.M. and Eapen V. (2014) Tourette Syndrome, disorder or spectrum? classificatory challenges and an appraisal of the DSM criteria. *Asian Journal of Psychiatry* , October 11 106–113 (doi: 10.1016/j.ajp.2014.05.010 (epub 2 June) .

Robertson M.M. and Eapen V. (2013). Wither the relationship between aetiology and phenotype in Tourette Syndrome. In: *Tourette Syndrome*; Eds Leckman J.F. and Martino D., Oxford University Press pages 361–394.

Rosenblatt, A. (2007) Neuropsychiatry of Huntington's disease. *Dialogues in Clinical Neuroscience*, 9 (2), 191–197.

Scahill, L., Erenberg, G., Berlin, C.M. *et al.* (2006) Contemporary assessment and pharmacotherapy of Tourette syndrome. *Journal of the American Society for Experimental NeuroTherapeutics*, 3, 192–206.

Scharf J.M., Yu D., Mathews C.A., Tourette Syndrome Association International Genetic Consortium, *et al.* (2012) Genome-wide association study of Tourette Syndrome. *Molecular Psychiatry* (epub August 14).

Vittori A. *et al.* (2014) Copy-number variation of the neuronal glucose transporter gene SLLC2A3 and age of onset in Huntington's disease. *Hum Mol Genet*, 23 (12), 3129–3137.

Chapter 31

Jones, R.N., Fong, T.G., Metzger, E. *et al.* (2010) Aging, brain disease, and reserve: implications for delirium. *American Journal of Geriatric Psychiatry*, 18 (2), 117–127.

Lyketsos, C.G., Kozauer, N. and Rabins, P.V. (2007) Psychiatric manifestations of neurologic disease: where are we headed? *Dialogues in Clinical Neuroscience*, 9 (2), 111–124.

Chapter 32

Bayley, J. (1998) *Iris*, Abacus, London.

Cardarelli, R., Kertesz, A., Knebl, J.A. (2010) Frontotemporal dementia: a review for primary care physicians. *American Family Physician*, 82 (11), 1372–1377.

Ihl, R., Frölich, L., Winblad, B. *et al.* (2011) World Federation of Societies of Biological Psychiatry (WFSBP) guidelines for the biological treatment of Alzheimer's disease and other dementias. *World Journal of Biological Psychiatry*, 12 (1), 2–32.

Katona, C., Livingston, G., Cooper, C. *et al.* (2007) International Psychogeriatric Association consensus statement on defining and measuring treatment benefits in dementia. *International Psychogeriatrics*, 19 (3), 345–354.

Livingston, G., Cooper, C., Woods, C. *et al.* (2008) Successful ageing in adversity. The LASER-AD longitudinal study. *Journal of Neurology, Neurosurgery and Psychiatry*, 79, 641–645.

Chapter 33

Bennett-Levy, J., Richards, D., Farrand, P. *et al.* (eds) (2010) *Oxford Guide to Low Intensity CBT Interventions*. Oxford University Press, Oxford.

Capriotti MR, Woods DW (2013) Cognitive-Behavioral Treatment for Tics. In: Martino D, Leckman JF (eds), Tourette Syndrome, Oxford University Press, Oxford, New York pp. 503–523.

Robins, C.J. and Chapman, A.L. (2004) Dialectical behavior therapy: current status, recent developments, and future directions. *Journal of Personality Disorders*, 18(1), 73–89.

Rollinson, R., Haig, C. and Warner, R. (2007) The application of cognitive-behavioral therapy for psychosis in clinical and research settings. *Psychiatric Services*, 58 (10), 1297–1302.

Chapters 34–37

Davis, J. (2006) The choice of drugs for schizophrenia. *New England Journal of Medicine*, 354, 518–520.

Kern, D. and Kumar, R. (2007) Deep brain stimulation. *Neurologist*, 13, 237–252.

Mann, J.J. (2005) The medical management of depression. *New England Journal of Medicine*, 353, 1819–1834.

Scott, A.I.F. (2005) College guidelines on electroconvulsive therapy: an update for prescribers. *Advances in Psychiatric Treatment*, 11, 150–156.

Taylor, D., Paton, C. and Kapur, S. (2009) *Maudsley Prescribing Guidelines*, 10th edn. Informa Healthcare, London.

Chapter 38

Lester, H. and Howe, A. (2008) Depression in primary care: three key challenges. *Postgraduate Medical Journal*, 84, 545–548.

Weich, S., Brugha, T., King, M. *et al.* (2011) Mental well-being and mental illness: findings from the Adult Psychiatric Morbidity Survey for England 2007. *British Journal of Psychiatry*, 199, 23–28.

Chapter 39

Coid, J.W. (2002) Personality disorders in prisoners and their motivation for dangerous and disruptive behaviour. *Criminal Behaviour and Mental Health*, 12 (3), 209–226.

Haque, Q. and Cumming, I. (2003). Intoxication and legal defences. *Advances in Psychiatric Treatment*, 9, 144–151.

Okai, D., Owen, G., Mcguire, H. *et al.* (2007) Mental capacity in psychiatric patients: systematic review. *British Journal of Psychiatry*, 191, 291–297.

Pompili, M., Lester, D., Innamorati, M. *et al.* (2009) Preventing suicide in jails and prisons: suggestions from experience with psychiatric inpatients. *Journal of Forensic Sciences*, 54 (5), 1155–1162.

Shaw, J., Hunt, I.M., Flynn, S. *et al.* (2006) Rates of mental disorder in people convicted of homicide: national clinical survey. *British Journal of Psychiatry*, 188, 143–147.

Völlm, B. (2009) Assessment and management of dangerous and severe personality disorders. *Current Opinion in Psychiatry*, 22 (5), 501–506.

Chapter 40

Candia, P.C. and Barba, A.C. (2011) Mental capacity and consent to treatment in psychiatric patients: the state of the research. *Current Opinion in Psychiatry* 24 (5), 442–446.

Department of Health (2008) Mental Capacity Act E-Learning Site, http://www.helpthehospices.org.uk/mca (accessed 16 February, 2012).

Chapters 41–43

Bamford Review of Mental Health and Learning Disability (N. Ireland) (2006) Internal papers and reports. http://www.rmhldni.gov.uk/index/internal-papers.htm (accessed 16 February, 2012).

Office of Public Sector Information (2007) Mental Health Act 2007, http://www.opsi.gov.uk/acts/acts2007/pdf/ukpga_20070012_en.pdf (accessed 16 February, 2012).

Office of Public Sector Information (2003) Mental Health (Care and Treatment) (Scotland) Act 2003, http://www.opsi.gov.uk/legislation/scotland/acts2003/20030013.htm (accessed 16 February, 2012).

Glossary

Affect: the observed external manifestation of emotion (see Chapter 2).

Affective disorder: mood disorder.

Agnosia: a loss of ability to recognise objects, people, sounds, smells or other sensory stimuli that is not due to sensory loss.

Akathisia: an unpleasant subjective feeling of restlessness resulting in an inability to sit still or a need to pace.

Anhedonia: inability to experience enjoyment when taking part in previously enjoyed activities.

Anxiety: subjective experience of worry or fear.

Arithmomania: a compulsion that involves counting (see Chapter 12).

Attention: the ability to focus selectively on a current task.

Automatic negative thoughts: thoughts that influence mood and behaviour and are experienced as coming unbidden into consciousness (e.g. 'They are probably not answering the phone because they hate me.'). Cognitive behavioural therapy is based on identifying and challenging such thoughts.

Avoidance: avoiding unpleasant thoughts or actual situations because they cause distress or anxiety.

Behavioural management: a system used to alter undesirable behaviour, usually employed in people with dementia or learning disability. The undesirable behaviour is analysed to determine its Antecedents (A), define the actual Behaviour (B) in detail and explore its Consequences (C). Practical interventions are then implemented to reduce it, and their success is monitored. For example, to reduce wandering in a person with dementia, an intervention may involve encouraging the carer to increase the amount of exercise the person has during the day and avoid them napping and taking caffeine.

Blunted affect: a patient's emotional response is very limited in range; the normal range of emotions (laughing or appearing sad at appropriate times) is not encountered; it is a negative symptom in schizophrenia.

Body dysmorphic disorder: an obsessional belief that parts of one's body are misshapen.

Care coordinator: member of the multidisciplinary team who is responsible for delivery of a patient's care. A coordinator reviews a patient regularly, organises Care Programme Approach meetings and ensures the care plan is carried out.

Care plan: a written treatment plan, usually agreed between health professionals and patients. It may include medication (and monitoring of it) and psychological and social interventions.

Care Programme Approach (CPA): the system by which patients of Community Mental Health Teams are managed through regular (at least six-monthly) meetings at which the patient and health professionals agree a care plan, which is then implemented by a care coordinator.

Catatonia: extreme disorder of motor function that occurs in catatonic schizophrenia; patients may stay still for hours; alternatively there may be periods of extreme motor activity. They may show stereotyped, repetitive movements, bizarre posturing, mutism, echolalia and echopraxia.

Chorea: rapid, jerky, dance-like movement of the body.

Circumstantial speech: speech that is discursive and takes a long time to get to the point.

Community Mental Health Team (CMHT): team of health and social care professionals who together deliver psychiatric services to people living in a defined area.

Compulsions: repetitive, purposeful, physical or mental behaviours performed with reluctance in response to an obsession. They are carried out according to certain rules in a stereotyped fashion and are designed to neutralise or prevent discomfort or a dreaded event.

Concentration: the ability to maintain attention on a current task. This is often tested in the cognitive examination by asking a patient to spell a word (e.g. 'world') backwards.

Confabulation: a falsified memory; patients with memory loss often confabulate because they cannot remember what has really happened.

Conversion: a synonym for dissociation (see below).

Core belief: central beliefs about oneself and the world that underlie thoughts and behaviours (see Chapter 33).

Counter-transference: the converse of transference, where the therapist experiences strong emotions towards the patient.

Defence mechanisms: psychological strategies employed unconsciously by people to reduce anxiety and feelings of internal conflict. Examples include splitting, denial and projection.

Deliberate self-harm: intentionally self-inflicted harm without a fatal outcome. The action may or may not have been carried out with the intent of causing death.

Delusion: fixed, false, firmly held belief out of keeping with the patient's culture and unaltered by evidence to the contrary. Types of delusion include grandiose delusions, persecutory delusions, thought insertion, withdrawal, broadcast, delusions of reference, passivity, somatic passivity, delusional perception and nihilistic delusions.

Delusional perception: a delusion that arises in response to a normal perception (see Chapter 6).

Delusions of grandiosity: a delusional belief that the patient has special abilities, powers or is an important person.

Delusions of guilt: a delusional belief that the patient has committed a terrible crime or other act. May occur in psychotic depression.

Delusions of jealousy/infidelity: a delusional belief that the patient's partner is being unfaithful.

Delusions of nihilism: a delusional belief that the patient has lost all their money, possessions or that they are dead or their body is rotting.

Delusions of persecution: a delusional belief that an organisation (e.g. MI5), person or other force is trying to harm the patient.

Psychiatry at a Glance, Sixth Edition. Cornelius Katona, Claudia Cooper, Mary Robertson. © 2016 John Wiley & Sons, Ltd. Published 2016 by John Wiley & Sons, Ltd.
Companion website: www.ataglanceseries.com/psychiatry

Delusions of reference: a delusional belief that events have a particular meaning to the patient (e.g. TV programmes are conveying messages, cars parked in the street are there for a special reason pertaining to the patient). The content is comparable to ideas of reference but they are held with delusional intensity.

Depersonalisation: the unpleasant experience of subjective change, feeling detached, unreal, empty within, unable to feel emotion, watching oneself from outside (e.g. 'It feels as if I am cut off by a pane of glass.').

Derealisation: the experience of the world or people in it seeming lifeless ('as if made out of cardboard').

Disinhibition: a loss of social conventions that leads to behaviour that is inappropriate to the social setting (e.g. overfamiliarity, type of clothing, sexual behaviour and speech).

Dissociative, dissociation: the process by which psychological distress is experienced as physical (usually in the form of neurological symptoms) (see Chapter 27).

Dual diagnosis: literally, fulfilling criteria for two diagnoses at once; in psychiatry this most often refers to the presence of a substance misuse disorder and a psychiatric disorder concurrently.

Dysmorphophobia: an excessive preoccupation with imagined or barely noticeable defects in physical appearance (e.g. preoccupation with the size of the nose, believing an objectively normal nose to be ugly and deformed).

Dysphasia: difficulty with understanding or verbally communicating. In cognitive assessments this is often tested by asking the patient to name objects and carry out a written command.

Dyspraxia: difficulty coordinating or performing purposeful movements and gestures in the absence of motor or sensory impairments. In cognitive assessments this is often tested by asking the patient to draw a clock face or two intersecting pentagons.

Echolalia: repeating words spoken by another person parrot-fashion.

Echopraxia: repeating the actions of another person.

Egodystonic: a thought that is experienced as troublesome and unwanted by the person experiencing it, who therefore tries to resist it. Obsessional thoughts are egodystonic.

Egosyntonic: a thought that is not experienced as unwanted or resisted.

Electroconvulsive therapy: treatment, usually for depression, that involves provoking seizures using controlled doses of electrical current applied through electrodes attached to the head (Chapter 37).

Expressed emotion: the quantity of critical and hostile comments and emotional overinvolvement displayed in relationships, typically within the family. A high level of expressed emotion in the home has been associated with a worse prognosis in people with schizophrenia.

Extrapyramidal symptoms: side effects of antipsychotic medication; includes Parkinsonian symptoms such as tremor, bradykinesia (slowness of movement) and akathisia (restlessness).

Flight of ideas: speech in which there is an abnormal connection between statements (see Chapter 2).

Flooding: type of behavioural therapy in which the patient is rapidly exposed to an anxiety-producing stimulus (Chapter 33).

Folie du pourquoi: the irresistible habit of seeking explanations for commonplace facts by asking endless questions (see Chapter 12).

Formal thought disorder: the patient's speech indicates that the links between consecutive thoughts are not meaningful; includes loosening of association.

Free association: the process in psychoanalysis whereby the patient is invited to say whatever comes into his or her mind.

Functional disorder: a psychiatric disorder in which there is no known physical cause (opposite of organic disorder).

Grandiosity: the patient's behaviour and speech indicate a belief that he or she is superior to others.

Habit reversal training: used in Tourette's syndrome, aims to increase awareness of tics and develop a competing response to them (e.g. relaxation).

Habituation: the decrease in anxiety that occurs with prolonged exposure to a situation that is initially anxiety-provoking (Chapter 33).

Hallucination: a perception in the absence of an external stimulus that is experienced as true and as coming from the outside world.

Hoarding: the acquisition of, and difficulty in discarding, items that appear worthless to others. Occurs in OCD and also in people without a psychiatric disorder.

Hypochondriasis: a preoccupation with health that is regarded as excessive by an observer. The ideas may be overvalued (exaggerated in degree or importance) or fully delusional.

Ideas of reference: thoughts that other people are looking at or talking about the patient, not held with full delusional intensity.

Illusion: distortion of a normal perception (e.g. interpreting a curtain cord as a snake).

Incongruous affect: emotion expressed by a patient differs markedly from that which might be expected in the situation (e.g. bright, happy affect while describing a painful bereavement).

Insight: the patient's understanding of his or her condition, its cause and the patient's willingness to accept treatment.

Korsakoff's psychosis: a cognitive disorder associated with thiamine deficiency usually due to chronic alcohol misuse, characterised by loss of short-term memory and confabulation. It usually follows Wernicke's encephalopathy (Chapter 18).

Learning theory: the theoretical basis for behavioural therapy, that people will be more likely to repeat actions that are associated with rewards (see operant conditioning).

Loosening of associations: speech in which there is no discernable link between statements (see Chapter 2).

Makaton: a communication system of signs and gestures used by some people with severe learning disabilities.

Mannerism: goal-directed, understandable movement (e.g. saluting).

Modelling: learning a behaviour by copying (e.g. people may be more likely to drink heavily if exposed regularly to a heavy drinking environment).

Mood: how a person is feeling in themselves; in the mental state the subjective mood (how the patient describes his or her feeling) and objective mood (the interviewer's assessment).

Morbid: a thought or feeling that is held with such intensity and is so preoccupying that it causes significant distress (e.g. morbid fear of fatness in eating disorders, morbid jealousy). The term may encompass delusions, obsessions and overvalued ideas.

Motivational interviewing: client-centred counselling that facilitates change by exploring ambivalence to that change; it is used to encourage establishment of healthy eating in eating disorders and to promote abstinence in substance use disorders.

Negative symptoms (of schizophrenia): symptoms characterised by the loss of normal functions, including lack of motivation, decreased thoughts and speech and social withdrawal.

Neologism: a made-up word (e.g. 'headshoe' to mean 'hat'); a second-rank symptom of schizophrenia.

Neuroleptic malignant syndrome: potentially fatal complication of antipsychotic treatment, involving hyperpyrexia, autonomic instability, confusion, increased muscle tone and raised serum creatine phosphokinase.

Neurosis: mental distress in which the ability to distinguish between symptoms originating from the patient's own mind and external reality is retained; includes most depressive and anxiety disorders.

Obsession: recurrent thoughts, feelings, images or impulses that are intrusive, persistent, senseless and/or unwelcome but are recognised as the patient's own.

Onomatomania: a compulsion that involves the desire to utter a socially unacceptable or inappropriate word (see Chapter 12).

Operant conditioning: the basic process by which an individual's behaviour is shaped by reinforcement or punishment; for example, alcohol consumption may be maintained by the rewards (reinforcement) of associated social life and pleasant feelings of relaxation and by punishment (unpleasant side effects) if a dependent drinker stops.

Organic disorder: psychiatric disorder with an identifiable physical cause (e.g. drug use, physical illness).

Orientation: awareness of the current day, date, time and year (orientation to time), location (orientation to place) and personal details, such as name and age (orientation to person).

Overvalued idea: an acceptable, comprehensible idea pursued by the patient beyond the bounds of reason and to an extent that causes distress to the patient or those around him or her.

Panic attack: discrete period of intense fear, impending doom or discomfort accompanied by characteristic somatic symptoms (see Chapter 11).

Perseveration: repeating words or topics.

Phobia: fear or anxiety that is out of proportion to the situation, cannot be reasoned or explained away and leads to avoidance behaviour.

Positive symptoms: the symptoms of schizophrenia characterised by abnormal thoughts and perceptions (i.e. hallucinations and delusions).

Premorbid personality: a description of the patient's character and attitudes before he or she became unwell (e.g. personality (whether sociable, short-tempered), hobbies and interests), which is given in the psychiatric history (see Chapter 1).

Pressure of speech: speech in which rate and volume are increased; it is usually difficult to interrupt.

Projection: a defence mechanism that involves attributing one's own feelings about something to others.

Pseudohallucination: perception in the absence of an external stimulus, experienced in internal space (i.e. inside one's head), with preserved insight.

Pseudoseizure: a seizure generated by the person deliberately or through subconscious processes rather than being due to electrical activity in the brain.

Psychiatric Intensive Care Unit (PICU): psychiatric inpatient ward with extra security, and higher staff/patient ratio, designed to manage patients who require additional security during their admission, usually owing to risk of violence or absconding.

Psychomotor agitation: an increase in overall motor activity; occurs in mania.

Psychomotor retardation: a decrease in overall motor activity; a sign of more severe depression.

Psychosis: severe mental disturbance characterised by a loss of contact with external reality. Delusions, hallucinations and disorganised thinking are often present.

Rapport: the interviewer's assessment of the warmth of relationship developed with the patient during an interview; it encompasses the extent of engagement and how forthcoming the patient was with information.

Rate of speech: the speed at which a person speaks; usually increased in mania and often decreased in depression.

Reciprocal inhibition: a technique in behavioural therapy that links desensitisation with a response incompatible with anxiety (e.g. relaxation, eating).

Rehabilitation psychiatry: branch of psychiatry concerned with recovery after serious psychiatric illness; there is usually a focus on psychological and social recovery.

Ritual: an action that has a 'magical' quality and is culturally sanctioned. This is not a psychiatric symptom but could potentially be confused with one by someone unfamiliar with the culture of the person performing the ritual.

Rumination: persistent preoccupation.

Somatic passivity: a delusion that an outside force is able to control one's bodily functions (e.g. generate sensations of heat or pain).

Somatisation: the experience of psychological distress as actual physical symptoms, often pain.

Splitting: a defence mechanism that involves separating in one's mind the positive and negative qualities of self and others so that people are perceived as all good or all bad.

Stereotypy: repetitive, purposeless movements (e.g. rocking in people with severe learning disability).

Suicide: intentional self-inflicted death.

Systematic desensitisation: graded exposure to a hierarchy of anxiety-producing situations.

Tardive dyskinesia: movements most often affecting the mouth, lips and tongue (e.g. rolling the tongue or licking the lips). They are usually the result of long-term administration of typical antipsychotics.

Thought block: a subjective experience that thoughts suddenly disappear (see Chapter 2).

Thought broadcasting: a delusional belief that one's thoughts are available to others; this may include the belief that they are being broadcast to everyone around or that they are known to specific people by a process similar to telepathy.

Thought echo: an auditory hallucination in which the patient hears his or her own thoughts spoken out loud.

Thought insertion: the patient experiences thoughts as being alien and not his or her own and therefore believes that they have been inserted by an external force.

Thought withdrawal: a delusional belief that the patient's thoughts are removed from his or her head by an external force.

Tic: a local and habitual twitching, especially in the face.

Transference: term given to an unconscious process in which a patient re-experiences strong emotions from early important relationships in his or her relationship with a therapist.

Index

Psychiatry at a Glance, Sixth Edition. Cornelius Katona, Claudia Cooper, Mary Robertson. © 2016 John Wiley & Sons, Ltd. Published 2016 by John Wiley & Sons, Ltd.
Companion website: www.ataglanceseries.com/psychiatry